The Health for All
policy framework
for the WHO European Region

2005 update

The World Health Organization was established in 1948 as the specialized agency of the United Nations responsible for directing and coordinating authority for international health matters and public health. One of WHO's constitutional functions is to provide objective and reliable information and advice in the field of human health. It fulfils this responsibility in part through its publications programmes, seeking to help countries make policies that benefit public health and address their most pressing public health concerns.

The WHO Regional Office for Europe is one of six regional offices throughout the world, each with its own programme geared to the particular health problems of the countries it serves. The European Region embraces some 880 million people living in an area stretching from the Arctic Ocean in the north and the Mediterranean Sea in the south and from the Atlantic Ocean in the west to the Pacific Ocean in the east. The European programme of WHO supports all countries in the Region in developing and sustaining their own health policies, systems and programmes; preventing and overcoming threats to health; preparing for future health challenges; and advocating and implementing public health activities.

To ensure the widest possible availability of authoritative information and guidance on health matters, WHO secures broad international distribution of its publications and encourages their translation and adaptation. By helping to promote and protect health and prevent and control disease, WHO's books contribute to achieving the Organization's principal objective – the attainment by all people of the highest possible level of health.

EUROPE

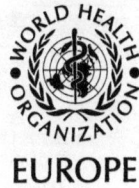

The Health for All
policy framework
for the WHO European Region

2005 update

European Health for All Series No. 7

WHO Library Cataloguing in Publication Data
The Health for All policy framework for the WHO European Region:
2005 update

(European Health for All Series; No. 7)

1.Health for All 2.Health policy 3.Health priorities 4.Regional health planning
5. Strategic planning 6.Europe I. Series

ISBN 92-890-1383-4   (NLM Classification : WA 540)
ISSN 1012-7356

ISBN 92-890-1383-4

Address requests about publications of the WHO Regional Office for Europe to:
Publications
WHO Regional Office for Europe
Scherfigsvej 8
DK-2100 Copenhagen Ø, Denmark
Alternatively, complete an online request form for documentation, health
information, or for permission to quote or translate, on the WHO/Europe web site
at http://www.euro.who.int/pubrequest.

Printed in Denmark

Contents

Foreword

This book presents the 2005 update of the Health for All policy framework for the WHO European Region, adopted at the fifty-fifth session of the WHO Regional Committee for Europe in September 2005. This is not a new policy but the third update of the Health for All strategy first approved by the Region in 1980. It reviews and reaffirms the previous update made in 1998 and known as HEALTH21, and incorporates the knowledge and experiences that have been accumulated since then. It also reflects the results of a wide consultation with Member States carried out in early 2005.

The 2005 update has been developed as a framework, not a users' manual, offering national policy-makers one possible architecture for a health policy – one based on values. It also reflects a broad consensus – that setting targets at the regional level does not take account of the overwhelming diversity in the social, economic and health status of the different countries in the Region. The 2005 update therefore does not include regional targets, while still strongly emphasising the usefulness of targets set at the national and subnational levels. Finally, the update strives to demonstrate that the Health for All values are not just abstract aspirations but that they can be implemented in practice. Pragmatic tools for policy-makers are presented that may enable them to test and check their national health policies, programmes and systems against the values commonly shared by society.

An open-ended Health for All process is suggested as a forum for exchanging information and experiences, generated at the national and subnational levels. Already a number of interesting ideas have come up during the consultation and in the discussions at the Regional Committee in September 2005. Countries have indicated special interest in more research; greater focus on the financial dimensions of Health for All policies; in-depth analysis of whether the functioning of health systems is linked to ethical, values-based governance; and the development of a set of benchmarks for the progressive implementation of Health for All and of concrete indicators for comparative analysis across countries.

Marc Danzon
Regional Director
WHO Regional Office for Europe

1. Background and rationale

Rationale

Ever since the WHO European Region launched its first regional Health for All strategy in 1980, it has committed itself to making periodic policy updates. These updates entail regular monitoring, evaluating, rethinking and revising of how the Region approaches and implements its Health for All policy.

An obligation – and an opportunity

On the one hand, the present update is mandatory – the WHO Regional Committee for Europe stipulated that the next update of the Region's Health for All policy be submitted in 2005 *(1)*. On the other hand, this obligation is also opportune – a good occasion to explore how the functioning of health systems is related to ethics and human rights. Moreover, this update gives us a chance to forge links between established WHO and Health for All concepts and public health policy-making at the beginning of the 21st century.

Consultation and guidance

The Tenth Standing Committee of the Regional Committee has been continuously involved in revisiting the European Region's Health for All policy framework. It has provided direction on the concept, process and methodology of the update. It suggested that the ethics of the health system be at the heart of this update and endorsed the core values that underpin Health for All and HEALTH21: *the health for all policy framework for the WHO European Region*, the 1998 update *(2)*. The Standing Committee also called for the current update to acknowledge changing political and economic circumstances and the growing need to translate values into guidelines and practical tools, despite the high complexity of such an endeavour. And finally, it urged elaboration of the concept of ethical governance as a novel way of linking values to implementation *(3)*.

The Regional Committee discussed this policy update at two sessions, before and during its preparation. At the fifty-third session, Member States agreed that the update should ensure continuity with HEALTH21 while reflecting new knowledge and recent developments, and that the core of the update should emphasize knowledge-based public health policies and the ethics of health systems *(4,5)*. The Regional Committee also approved the methodology and approach to be taken by the Regional Office in preparing the update. Member States were then given a progress report at the fifty-fourth session *(6)*.

Approach and methodology

The Regional Office has also regarded the present update as an opportunity. It initiated the process early, to allow ample collaboration and consultation with Member States. In 2003, when work began, the Regional Office decided that it made sense to develop the document along three analytical axes. They comprise the three main pillars of the update, each answering one core question.

Pillar one: How has Health for All policy influenced policy-making in the Member States?
The European Observatory on Health Systems and Policies responded to this question by conducting a comprehensive overview of how the Health for All policy has been used in the European Region. To do so, the Observatory initiated two studies in 2003. The first study provides a synopsis of the de facto adoption and use of Health for All concepts in Member States. The second study, still under way at the time of publication of this update, assesses countries' experiences with health target programmes and describes the design and implementation of national health targets. Some of the studies' findings are presented in Chapter 4.

Pillar two: What are the Health for All values that underpin and drive policy-making?
To help answer this question, an international think-tank was assembled, consisting of experts with broad knowledge and experience in

formulating, assessing and implementing health policies internationally, nationally and subnationally. The main challenges for the group were:

- to identify and describe the values that play a role in health decision-making and are widely accepted throughout the Region, taking account of the varying contexts in which they occur;
- to develop definitions of these common values in order to better understand them pragmatically and ethically;
- to link these values to the factors that shape health policies and actions;
- to review international legal frameworks (existing international human rights instruments, such as conventions, declarations and treaties) for these values; and
- to elaborate a vision of ethical governance in health as a way to translate these values into action.

Their conclusions are presented in Chapter 5.

Pillar three: How can Health for All values be put into practice?
To address this question, a review was conducted of available tools that might enable decision-makers to construct national Health for All policies and programmes. A wide range of such tools already exists in many countries. While they have not been explicitly developed to implement or assess values, they can be used to do so. From the tools reviewed, 10 main types were chosen to exemplify the possibilities. The selection was based on whether a given type had proven useful at a national level, was holistic and adaptable, had been tested, was undergoing further improvement and was available. The methodology and the suggested tools are presented in Chapter 6.

Finally, Chapter 7 offers policy-makers some guidelines for determining how well their own national health policies promote Health for All.

What this update is – and is not
This update of the European Health for All policy framework has been developed to be inspiring rather than prescriptive. It does not provide a model for Member States to adopt or emulate, but merely offers a possible architecture for health policy – one that is based on a

particular vision and values. In developing their own policies, countries are invited to use this framework in whatever way seems most useful, adapting it to their specific health, economic, cultural and historical needs. Ultimately, the true determinant of success is how an individual country approaches such a process, and policy-makers must decide for themselves which Health for All elements their national health policy will incorporate. In other words, the present update is meant to be a framework that encourages choice.

For example, each country must decide itself whether to allocate specific funds for implementing the Health for All vision. Where financial resources are limited, such allocation might be used as a tool to ensure that the Health for All values are respected within the health sector. However, the adoption of such a financial tool must be country-specific, and a recommendation cannot be made at the regional level. Another national choice to make is whether to adopt one single domestic Health for All policy, or to integrate Health for All into every existing national policy that has an impact on health, to ensure that it respects the Health for All values and conforms to the concept of ethical governance.

It is important to emphasize that the present document is only an update of the European Health for All policy framework, not a new policy. Only seven years have passed since the adoption of HEALTH21. The Standing Committee of the Regional Committee felt that, given the relatively short time that has elapsed, it was premature to develop and propose an entirely new policy for the Region *(3)*.

Target-setting has been a traditional approach in the European Region's Health for All policy formulation. Recently, however, there has been a consensus that establishing common targets for all countries in the Region can often be artificial, unfair or simply uninspiring. It does not take into account significant differences in Member States' public health and economic development. Nonetheless, setting targets can be an important exercise at national and sometimes subnational levels. National targets can be an excellent implementation and guidance tool, as well as a means for a country to articulate its degree of ambition.

And when all stakeholders are involved, the formulation of national health targets can help ensure their joint ownership of health policy.

The recommendations included in this update are not exhaustive, nor do they cover every field of public health. Instead, the focus is on fields and methods that are either new or have evolved significantly since 2000. Even though HEALTH21 was adopted a short time ago, the intervening period has seen many significant changes in the health systems of Member States. Some of the experience and knowledge they have acquired is presented here.

In other words, rather than attempting to produce an authoritative document that finalizes the Region's Health for All policy, this update aims to encourage an open-ended Health for All process. The Health for All policy framework can then be continuously enriched by the broad range of Health for All activities that individual countries themselves choose to carry out. Some countries may decide to develop and analyse national case studies. Other Member States may regard this update as an invitation to re-examine and revisit their health policies. Still others might devote special attention to the communications challenge – how best to communicate the Health for All values, the concept of health and human rights, and the model of ethical governance to different audiences and stakeholders. There may also be countries that elect to develop concrete benchmarks against which to measure the implementation of Health for All policies. Meanwhile, a given country might focus on the local level because it sees decentralization and the meeting of local health needs as essential in successfully implementing Health for All. Finally, a group of countries could invest effort in developing national and subnational health targets and linking them to the United Nations Millennium Development Goals (MDGs).

Most of these ideas were suggested by individual countries during consultation on the present update. They are only a few among many possible national activities and developments that could help give the European Health for All process a new, open-ended dynamic. The process could serve as a forum for exchanging up-to-date health policy information, experiences and ideas. National and subnational updates could in turn contribute elements and ideas to the continuing evolution of the regional Health for All policy, in a permanent process of renewal and improvement. Such a development would be the best testament to this document's relevance and usefulness. It is also hoped that the present update will serve as a valuable tool for promoting the ethical development of health policies.

Continuity with related initiatives

Continuity with HEALTH21

The Health for All movement in the WHO European Region has been marked by continuity, and the present update is the latest step in a cumulative development. Since its adoption in 1998, HEALTH21 has met with wide acceptance throughout the Region. That framework update conveyed a broad vision of public health, underpinned by the core values of the global Health for All movement, and it outlined the general approach and direction that individual countries might take. It remains valid, and the present update reaffirms HEALTH21 as the broad policy framework that guides the work of the Regional Office in its support for Member States.

The 2005 update upholds and reinforces the values, basic principles, coverage and vision of HEALTH21. Specifically, it reiterates the following key principles underpinning the framework.

- The ultimate goal of health policy is to achieve the full health potential of everyone.
- Closing the health gap between and within countries (i.e. solidarity) is essential for public health in the Region.
- People's participation is crucial for health development.
- Health development can be achieved only through multisectoral strategies and intersectoral investments that address health determinants.
- Every sector of society is accountable for the health impact of its own activities.

In particular, the update addresses HEALTH21's call to "provide up-to-date evidence-based tools that countries can use to turn policies based on health for all into action". And finally, it reiterates the significance of the 21 HEALTH21 targets because "they provide a framework for the Region as a whole, and an inspiration for the construction of targets at the country and local levels". HEALTH21 describes its own set of targets by saying they are not meant to be prescriptive, but that together they make up the essence of the regional policy *(7)*. The present update maintains this flexible approach.

In short, the current document amplifies HEALTH21's role as "fundamentally, a charter for social justice, providing a science-based guide to better health development and outlining a process that will lead to progressive improvement in people's health".

Consistency with other major health policy strategies

The present Health for All update is also consistent with other major health policy formulations. For instance, the update has been developed in parallel with **WHO's Eleventh General Programme of Work**, which is currently being prepared and will, when adopted in 2006, outline the main directions for the Organization's work through 2015. The two documents share a number of key characteristics, notably a common foundation in core WHO and Health for All values, a reaffirmation of the guiding role these values play in WHO work, a particular focus on the rights and needs of vulnerable populations, and a flexible approach to national circumstances in the implementation of policy.

This update is also strongly linked to several of the Regional Office's key policies. In particular, its recognition of the need for a country-specific approach to health and for national interpretation and implementation of Region-wide concepts supports the vision espoused by the **Regional Office's Country Strategy "Matching services to new needs"** *(8)*. The Health for All update and the Country Strategy are also united in their call for developing partnerships outside the health sector. Moreover, in consonance with the next phase of the Country Strategy – focused on strengthening health systems – this update places strong emphasis on health systems as the appropriate setting for national Health for All efforts.

Finally, the update is also consistent with the position taken by the Regional Office on the United Nations MDGs (9). The values of equity, solidarity and participation at the centre of the Health for All update also lie at the heart of the Regional Office's MDG strategy. These three values are especially significant due to the economic heterogeneity of the Region, in which poverty continues to require a great deal of attention – not only in low- and middle-income countries but also in the richest countries. These values are highlighted by the MDG strategy's emphasis on two problems – how to achieve the MDGs in countries where they are unlikely to be met, and how to identify from the national aggregate data in individual countries the vulnerable subpopulations that the MDGs are most relevant to, and then direct efforts accordingly.

2. The history of Health for All

The global Health for All movement
The 1946 Constitution of the World Health Organization states that "the health of all peoples is fundamental to the attainment of peace and security" (10). The Constitution also recognizes "the enjoyment of the highest attainable standard of health" as a fundamental human right. By the late 1970s, the widespread enjoyment of this right was still far from being achieved, with about one thousand million people in the world living in such poverty that acceptable standards of health were impossible. Recognizing the challenge, WHO and its Member States set about creating a framework to help translate the vision of universal health into a strategy and policy. The process began in 1977 with a call for national governments and WHO to work towards one goal: to enable all of the world's citizens to enjoy by 2000 a level of health that would allow them to lead a socially active and economically productive life (11). This vision and movement have come to be known as Health for All.

The Health for All concept was subsequently introduced at the 1978 International Conference on Primary Health Care in Alma-Ata (in the former USSR). The Declaration of Alma-Ata states that attaining health for all as part of overall development starts with primary health care based on "acceptable methods and technology made universally accessible to individuals and families in the community through their full participation and at a cost that the community and the country can afford" (12).

Since then, Member States have been urged to consider the Health for All concept when formulating policies and action plans. It was believed that, by interpreting Health for All in a national social, political and developmental context, each country would be able to contribute to the global aim of health for all by the year 2000.

The call for health for all was, and fundamentally remains, a call for social justice, equity and solidarity, and a societal response that strives for unity in diversity. Rather than enshrining a single finite goal, Health for All is instead a process of bringing countries to progressive improvement in the health of all their citizens. Globally, WHO has continued to pursue its own commitment to health for all, by:

- adopting in 1981 the Global Strategy for Health for All by the Year 2000 *(13)* and approving, one year later, a global action plan for implementing the Strategy *(14)*;
- renewing the Health for All strategy in 1995 *(15)* by developing a holistic health policy – still based on equity and solidarity but with further emphasis on individual, family and community responsibility for health – and by placing health within an overall development framework;
- linking the renewed strategy to programme budgets and evaluation *(16)*; and
- launching in 1999, after consultation with and within the Member States, a global Health for All policy for the 21st century *(17)*.

Health for All in the European Region
In 1980, the Regional Committee for Europe approved a European strategy for attaining health for all by the year 2000 *(18)*. It decided to monitor the strategy's implementation every two years (beginning in 1983), and to evaluate its effectiveness every six years (beginning in 1985).

Following the initial launch of a European Health for All policy, the Regional Committee asked for the formulation of specific regional targets to assist in implementation of the regional strategy. Such targets were thought necessary in order to motivate and actively involve Member States in committing to Health for All. The first Health for All policy and targets in support of the regional strategy were adopted in 1984 *(19)*. They provided a broad but precisely drawn vision of health development in the Region. They also outlined a clear ethical framework for policy development – instead of focusing solely on inputs to health services (characteristic of an inward-looking, hospital-oriented health sector), they also emphasized outcomes, encouraging a shift to a health sector that reaches out and is oriented towards primary care. In addition, a list of 65 indicators, linked to the 38 regional targets, was devised to measure progress.

In the same year, the Regional Committee also adopted an action plan for implementing the regional strategy. This described the roles and actions to be taken by Member States, the Regional Committee and the Regional Office, respectively. While the plan was again directly linked to the regional targets, it also left room for each country to define its own priorities and strategies.

With the adoption of these three documents in 1984, the Regional Committee created a framework for health policies in the Region. At the same time, it also established a mechanism to regularly monitor and evaluate progress towards achieving health for all in the Region by 2000. As a consequence of this commitment, an update of the regional policy, strategy and targets was made in 1991 *(20)*. Meanwhile, the Regional Committee also assessed progress towards the regional targets every three years, in 1985, 1988, 1991, 1994 and 1997.

In 1998, a revised European Health for All policy framework, entitled HEALTH21, was adopted *(1)*. It reflected the extraordinary changes that had occurred in the Region since the previous regional policy, including the addition of 20 new pluralistic societies and their emerging voices, as well as, despite many positive developments, severe economic downturns that had led to major crises in the health sector. HEALTH21 articulates two primary aims, three basic values and four main strategies. Its 21 targets also provide benchmarks to measure progress in improving and protecting health and in reducing health risks.

3. Main characteristics of a Health for All policy

A health policy that can be described as a Health for All policy has several key features. This chapter briefly summarizes these characteristics.

Values-based and values-driven

Health for All is and has always been about values, and the Health for All policy framework links a set of basic values to the development of health policy. Among them, the core Health for All value is equity. In the Health for All context, equity means that everyone has a fair opportunity to attain his or her full health potential.

A concern for equity has direct implications for how decision-makers choose their priorities in health policy – how they decide which public health issues and which population groups merit the most attention. Health policies built on concern for equity will ensure that health services are fairly distributed within the population. This means that priority is given to the poor and other vulnerable and socially marginalized groups. Health systems based on equity contribute to the empowerment and social inclusion of such disadvantaged groups.

Health for All also incorporates the closely linked value of solidarity, which is usually interpreted as a society's sense of collective responsibility. In Health for All contexts, solidarity means that everyone contributes to the health system according to his or her ability. Solidarity can be seen as a way to ensure equity. A health policy that promotes solidarity is better able to counterbalance the unequal impact of health determinants on access to services and health outcomes. In contrast, a health policy that does not value solidarity will typically privilege those who are already wealthy, more educated and more proactive in taking advantage of health care entitlements.

Equity and solidarity are directly linked to a third value that has become increasingly important in the Health for All movement – participation. The active participation of health system stakeholders, including both individuals and organizations, improves the quality of public health decision-making.

These three values of equity, solidarity and participation directly affect health system financing, access to health services, efforts to improve population health and the development of high-quality programmes in the sector. They also affect the dissemination of health information, since the uneven dissemination of information contributes to inequity and, conversely, information sharing is an important tool in combating it. While there will always be a need to pitch some health communications to the general population, focus on particular, individual lifestyle choices and behaviours should not undermine the importance of public health policies and structural, intersectoral initiatives. Respect for core societal values – or a lack thereof – affects such policies and initiatives as much as it does the population served.

Health for All employs a broad vision of health

In the Preamble to the WHO Constitution, health is described as "a state of complete physical, mental and social well-being and not merely the absence of disease or infirmity". Health for All amplifies this vision of health even further.

A broad vision within the health sector

In accordance with the Health for All policy framework, a health policy should address more than just patient care. Today, this belief appears to be widespread, especially in countries that have adopted and developed national Health for All policies. Nevertheless, policy-makers throughout the European Region often find it difficult to incorporate other elements in their health policies. In several countries, these policies revolve chiefly around health care. Though the Health for

All framework recognizes that the quality of patient care contributes significantly to a population's health status, it regards care as only one of many factors in health improvement. Other major influences include the variety of social and economic circumstances in which people live and work. There is ample evidence that these structural determinants of population health play a key role in this rapidly changing Region. That is why the Health for All framework calls for policy-makers to look beyond health care and recommends a better policy balance among all the key factors that contribute to population health. In a Health for All policy, such a balance will be necessarily reflected in the budget allocations. This is in tune with some countries' efforts to improve the effectiveness of disease-specific programmes by adopting a more general approach to strengthening their national health systems.

In the Health for All vision, four types of programme efforts contribute to health improvement.

- **Patient care** is an essential but not exclusive element of a Health for All approach.
- **Prevention** includes activities such as immunizations, health surveillance and early detection programmes, all of which tend to be well integrated into routine health care.
- **Promotion of healthy lifestyles** addresses issues such as nutrition, exercise and the consumption of tobacco, alcohol and other drugs. The need to promote healthy lifestyles is widely recognized, but often only in an abstract way. When it comes to making health promotion part of policy and funding it, progress can be quite slow.
- **Addressing health determinants** is an area closely related to health promotion, but it goes beyond individual behaviour to tackle aspects of the physical, social and economic environment that affect health, most notably poverty. Actions addressing health determinants include legislation, policy-setting and cross-sector advocacy (see Box 1).

In order for policy-making to be as informed and balanced as possible, Health for All emphasizes the importance of giving health professionals

---

BOX 1. ADDRESSING HEALTH DETERMINANTS

One area that demands action in addressing health determinants is environmental health. Most countries recognize its importance, but their awareness does not translate consistently into practice. A general commitment to environmental health is not enough; the best results arise from strong public awareness and a political determination to act.

Another important area is poverty. Since poverty is a major source of health inequity, a Health for All policy should address poverty reduction, ensuring that the health system is responsive to poor, marginal and vulnerable population groups. From a Health for All perspective, action on poverty and other health determinants is considered properly intersectoral, with the health sector playing a leading role.

---

a role in discussing, evaluating and improving health policies. Most health professionals are primarily involved in direct provision of health care, and they can not only bring medical knowledge and skills to the policy process but also add credibility. Some of them can also provide advice from experience in other health activities (such as nursing and health promotion).

A broad vision beyond the health sector

In the Health for All vision, health improvement is not the exclusive responsibility of the health sector. There are far too many examples of how other sectors' policies can lead to an increase in poor health that the health sector must then address. Such problems can be avoided by involving other sectors in health improvement. Tobacco, alcohol and nutrition are just three examples of issues on which it is advantageous for the health sector to collaborate with other sectors, such as environment, education, agriculture and industry. Working intersectorally enhances efficiency and provides many additional opportunities for health interventions. For instance, health system development should be placed high on local, regional and national development agendas, rather than confined solely to the health sector as an item of public expenditure.

Healthier people have greater human capital, and therefore the health sector has significant potential to impact the overall development and economic growth of a country. This interaction between health and other sectors is a two-way process.

Non-health professionals, such as teachers or economists, can also play an important role in health issues. However, it is important to remember that such professionals are often just the most visible elements of other sectors that impact health, so values such as equity in health need to be linked to the entire structure of each of these sectors.

Health systems as the setting for Health for All

Health systems are societal institutions and, as such, their development needs to be based on and driven by values. For a national health system to be consistent with the Health for All vision and values, it must have several important features (21).

- **Universal availability**. There should be enough functioning health and public health facilities, goods and services to meet the needs of everyone in the country. Programme capacities should be similarly sufficient. The determination of what is necessary for a particular country depends on the national context and level of development.

- **Universal accessibility**. The need for accessibility applies to every element of the health sector, but it is particularly critical for primary care. Access has an economic dimension (affordability), a geographical dimension (physical accessibility), an ethical and human rights dimension (accessibility to all population groups equally, without discrimination) and a communications dimension (accessibility of information).

- **Universal acceptability**. All health facilities, goods and services, including communication and information, should be culturally appropriate and respectful of cultural differences and traditions.

- **Quality improvement**. Mechanisms to ensure the continuous improvement and upgrading of health services have become increasingly important to Health for All policies. The benefits of such changes should be evenly distributed among all social groups, not just available to those who can pay for them. Quality improvement efforts should focus on how much particular changes can improve health. For instance, adopting procedures that ensure patient safety is one efficient way to boost quality. The benefits of quality improvement include better health, improved relations between the general public and health professionals, and a decrease in costly failures in patient treatment.

In Europe, health systems can be described as having three essential goals – health gain, fairness and responsiveness. All three are in harmony with the Health for All concept. Improved health is not only an end in itself but also a major factor for overall development, which is another reason why health gains should be equally distributed among all population groups. Fairness in financial contributions to health requires that there be sufficient funding to enable universal access to health services without forcing individuals or families into poverty. A health system that is driven by Health for All goals should also respond to the non-medical expectations of both individuals and society, for instance by safeguarding patient dignity, confidentiality and autonomy; respecting patient rights; being sensitive to the specific needs and vulnerabilities of all population groups; and promoting social inclusion and poverty reduction. Finally, a health system that respects Health for All is efficient, by producing the best health outcomes from available resources.

The way a health system works reflects ethical choices. This is true for the four core functions of a health system – provision of services, financing, resource generation, and stewardship and governance. Of these, the biggest challenge to solidarity and equity lies in how a health system is financed. In a system based on the Health for All values, budgets should be drawn up to reflect the relative contributions of the various budget items to health improvement. For example, a policy that favours sophisticated high-technology investments should make sure that all population groups benefit.

Health in all policies

The Health for All concept calls for a broad partnership approach to health. The Regional Office for Europe works with a range of international partners, including the Council of Europe, the World Bank, the European Commission, nongovernmental organizations and private partners. This cooperation helps ensure that the support the Regional Office provides to individual countries is consistent with that provided by other public health stakeholders. Such a collaborative approach also makes better health outcomes possible by uniting the forces of disparate partners and setting common agendas, while exploiting each one's specific strengths and capabilities. With regard to the Health for All policy framework, such synergy is essential.

The European Region shares certain common societal values, and respect for these values is seen in the policies and actions of all international stakeholders. A good example is the work done within the European Union (EU) system. Through its legal and financial mechanisms, the EU has achieved a great deal in public health throughout the WHO European Region. For instance, not only are environmental standards now enshrined in EU legislation, they are also automatically applied to countries joining the EU and used as reference standards by neighbouring countries. In addition, numerous EU institutions contribute to health-related activities, such as the European development banks and the European Commission with their Public Health, TACIS (Technical Assistance to the Commonwealth of Independent States) and Phare programmes *(22)*. In general, EU legislation strengthens the cause of health in every policy that affects the social and economic development of its Member States.

A common ground of shared values makes international partnerships for health easier to initiate and sustain. At present, the Health for All concept and values permeate a variety of the European Region's technical policies; they also characterize the commitments that Member States have made before the Regional Committee (see Annex 1). It would be a great step forward for the Region if the major stakeholders in public health were to enshrine in policy the concept of ethical, values-based governance (see Chapter 6).

4. Health for All in the countries of the WHO European Region

This chapter presents the findings of an exploratory study carried out by the European Observatory on Health Systems and Policies in 2003–2004. It analysed the influence of the Health for All concept on the national health policies of the 52 Member States in the WHO European Region. (Subnational policies, which were included to reflect the process of decentralization being pursued in some countries, are described separately below.) For the purposes of this study, a national health policy was classified as a Health for All policy if it satisfied four criteria:

- it commits itself to the goal of health for all in a document
- it introduces a multisectoral perspective
- it is explicitly values-oriented
- it includes health targets.

The study methodology included documentary analysis, a literature review, country case studies and interviews with experts. Its main findings are summarized below.

- The European Health for All policy framework has influenced the formulation of most Member State health policies.

- The framework's role in national health policy-making has ranged from no influence to source of inspiration to blueprint.

- The core Health for All values have been broadly accepted throughout the Region.

- At the same time, almost every country has taken its own approach, most notably in setting its own national health targets.

- There remains a large gap between Health for All policy formulation and actual implementation.

Health for All policies in Member States

National and subnational policies

Of the 52 health policies analysed, 40 policies satisfy all four Health for All criteria listed above. Nine of the qualifying ones exist only as draft health policies, though some Member States that are currently drafting such policies previously had other Health for All policies in place. Among the 12 Member States without qualifying policies, 2 have sectoral health policy documents that satisfy all the criteria except multisectorality. The Russian Federation provides a unique example: it has issued a number of Health for All policy papers focusing on single sectors (notably health care delivery).

Subnational Health for All policy documents were identified in 22 Member States, but it should be noted that the data on them are not as complete as for national policies. Some countries that have not formulated national Health for All policies have subnational policies, and vice versa. The vast majority of the countries have Health for All policies on at least one level.

Timetables

A Health for All policy timetable runs from its start date to its end date, when its health targets are supposed to have been achieved. Thirty-six of the Health for All documents start between 1994 and 2003. Most of the timetables cover 7 to 10 years. The shortest lasts 3 years, while some last 20 years. In three cases, the endpoint of the timetable is indefinite. In 11 policy documents, the health targets have several end dates rather than a single one.

Policy continuity and discontinuity

Many Member States have shown lasting interest in formulating Health for All policies. Twenty-seven Member States formulated Health for

All policies prior to their most recent efforts. The form this continuing commitment takes may or may not change over time, as the examples in Boxes 2–4 illustrate.

BOX 2. FINLAND: CONTINUITY IN BOTH POLICY FORMULATION AND STRATEGIC FOCUS

Finland is a case study in making a commitment to Health for All that appears to be unaffected by political changes. Its 1987 Health for All policy was subsequently reviewed, evaluated and revised. After its end date, a new policy building on the previous experiences was formulated in 2001 *(23–25)*.

BOX 3. THE UNITED KINGDOM: CONTINUITY IN POLICY FORMULATION AND A SHIFT IN STRATEGIC FOCUS

The Health of the Nation policy launched in 1992 was suspended after the 1997 general election. Evaluation of the policy revealed a number of weaknesses: key actors questioned the credibility and relevance of the targets, a lack of ownership was reported, and the policy had no effect on resource allocation. Despite these deficiencies, the government chose to retain a health policy approach and gave England, Northern Ireland, Scotland and Wales each the responsibility for developing its own policy. In comparing the resultant four new policies with the previous national policy, a clear change in emphasis becomes evident: equity and health determinants have now gained a prominent place *(26,27)*.

BOX 4. GERMANY: A GAP IN POLICY FORMULATION

Following the Member States' adoption of the first European Health for All policy, the Federal Republic of Germany was inspired to try to devise its own Health for All policy. The Minister of Health coined the slogan "Cost containment is not enough" and commissioned a report on priority health problems. The report was published in 1987 and republished in 1990, after reunification, to incorporate material on the eastern part of the country (the former German Democratic Republic) *(28,29)*. Despite its merits and unchallenged quality, the report was criticized for its political approach. The Health for All approach was alleged to be inadequate for industrialized countries, and it was argued, moreover, that with its targets a Health for All policy resembled a socialist economic plan. It took almost 10 years before the Federal Ministry of Health launched a new initiative to formulate a policy with targets, drawing on contributions by 70 institutions and more than 200 health care and public health experts. Eventually, in 2003, the policy was adopted as the German health target document *(30)*.

Policy enforcement and legal status

Among the 40 Health for All policies analysed, 35 are set out in official documents, while 5 are published as unofficial reports (see Table 1).

Table 1. European national Health for All policies, by status and document type

Status	Document type		Total
	Official	Unofficial	
In force	28	3	31
Draft	7	2	9
Total	35	5	40

The source of the documents generally indicates who has had the lead role in developing the policy. Usually it is either the government or the competent ministry, but in two instances the legislature was involved, and in one the head of state took the opportunity to associate the policy with his leadership.

The legal standing of the various Health for All policies varies widely. Some countries make their health policies law, as France did by swiftly adopting into law a policy that had taken a long time to develop. In Italy, the national Health for All policy has a strong binding character – although it has not been politically endorsed in legislation, it constitutes an important reference framework for many national policy documents, such as the National Health Plan and the report on the health status of the Italian population.

Some countries have approved their policy by decree in order to underline its importance. In 2003, the Parliament of Sweden adopted a national Health for All public health policy to deal with all major health determinants. This put public health higher on the political agenda, and a special minister for public health was appointed. In addition, a government bill gave the Swedish National Institute for Public Health a special role in implementing the country's public health policy. In 1998, the Grand National Assembly of Turkey formally adopted the European Health for All framework policy, expressing a clear commitment to it by a national programme that includes an action plan through to 2020.

From this programme, 10 specific national health goals have been formulated.

For a number of Member States, an official document would be a rather unfamiliar way to formulate a policy. The policy instrument that comes closest is the white paper, used by governments in the United Kingdom and elsewhere to lay out a policy or proposed policy. Usually a white paper signifies the government's clear intention to make a policy law. Other methods used to indicate policy intentions include party programmes and election platforms. However, no matter what form they take, such intentions often get lost when political conditions change.

Policy statements that provide orientation without obligation are considered "soft law". Even when they play no role in drafting legislation, they can still motivate and inspire, though the question remains as to whether their non-binding status is a good thing. The answer varies from situation to situation.

The particular form that a Health for All policy document takes may also reflect who is promulgating it. Political responsibility for Health for All can rest with the head of government, the cabinet or the competent minister. In principle, the head of government usually determines major policy directions, the cabinet decides government policy and the ministers implement it, but these roles can vary considerably.

Finally, it should be noted that a health policy may take a specific form for reasons of political expediency, such as to strengthen alliances, secure political legitimacy or facilitate implementation.

The values
HEALTH21 describes three core values: health as a fundamental human right; equity in health and solidarity in action; and participation and accountability. Of the 40 national Health for All policies identified in the Observatory study, 20 policies refer explicitly to all three values, 12 policies to two, 6 policies to just one and 2 to none at all. To consider it from another angle, 25 of the policies refer specifically to health as

a human right, 34 to equity and solidarity and 31 to participation and accountability.

The evidence strongly shows that the values formulated in HEALTH21 are present in national health policy documents developed before HEALTH21 was drafted. This suggests that these values are not any innovation of HEALTH21, but rather that HEALTH21 shares the European Region's general ethical orientation.

Health targets

The European Region proposed 38 targets in its first Health for All policy in 1984 and again in the 1991 update, while in the 1998 update, HEALTH21, it suggests 21 targets. In the 40 Health for All policies analysed, the number of targets range from 4 to 100. Eight policies exceed the 38 targets proposed in the 1984 policy, and 16 policies have more than the 21 targets of HEALTH21. Four Member States have adopted every HEALTH21 target word for word.

It has been argued that in setting health targets, the trend is to be more pragmatic, focusing on only a few targets because of the difficulty in attaining a large number of them. However, the evidence for this observation is not clear, and even in cases where only a few targets are defined, the subtargets can be quite numerous.

Member States have usually chosen HEALTH21 targets that match the technical focus of their policies. Analysis of the targets in the 40 national Health for All policies reveals some interesting points.

- Three targets appear in three quarters of the policies: "Improving mental health", "Healthier living" and "Reducing harm from alcohol, drugs and tobacco".

- Three targets appear in less than a quarter of the policies: "Solidarity for health in Europe", "Mobilizing partners for health" and "Policies and strategies for health for all".

- Member States have adjusted many HEALTH21 targets to reflect their individual needs and circumstances.

- Some national policies also introduce health targets not yet covered by Health for All, reflecting particular national and subnational priorities.

How has the European Health for All policy influenced the formulation of national health policies?

Self-reported influence

The most obvious indicator of the overall influence of the European Health for All policy on national health policies is the impact mentioned in the policy documents themselves. Of the 40 Health for All policies analysed 32 documents explicitly refer to the European Health for All policy as a framework or source of inspiration; 14 of these documents mention a policy version from 1991 or earlier, 14 mention HEALTH21 (1998) and 4 both; and 6 documents cite the involvement of WHO experts in the drafting process.

The national Health for All policy documents from eight countries do not show any explicit link to the European Health for All policy: Belarus, Denmark, Estonia, France, Ireland, Italy, the Netherlands and The former Yugoslav Republic of Macedonia.

Translating the European policy framework into a national context

The previous sections described evidence of similarities between the European and the national Health for All policy documents. In addition, the study also examined causality: have national health policies really been influenced by the European Health for All framework, and if so, through what means? Three mechanisms were identified.

- **Policy transfer.** A country or subnational entity can intentionally adopt a health policy originally developed somewhere else. The transfer may include institutional structures, ideologies, attitudes and ideas. Policy transfers can involve direct copying into legislation, though the existence of Health for All elements does not necessarily mean that a WHO Health for All policy was the model (see Box 5, for example).

BOX 5. POLICY TRANSFER IN KAZAKHSTAN – A DIRECT LINK

After gaining independence in 1991, Kazakhstan sought to adopt a Health for All policy. The country needed a new health policy for a number of reasons: economic difficulties inherent in the transition to independence, deteriorating population health and an urgent need to address the issue of poverty and equity in health. Moreover, there were fundamental problems in the way the old health system was functioning. Reforms were needed to transform it from a hospital-based service to one that was more oriented toward primary care, and to introduce a multisectoral public health approach that included health promotion. Finally, several urgent health problems had to be addressed, including environmental issues such as the radioactive and toxic chemical sites associated with the former defence industries, the drying up of the Aral Sea and the heavily polluted industrial east. The Health for All model enabled the country to confront these issues, and WHO experts were involved in drafting the policy from the early stages. During the process, a consensus arose to position the Kazakh health policy in a wider political context under government stewardship. Health now forms a part of the general strategic policy, called Kazakhstan 2030, and the president has endorsed the country's Health for All policy.

- **Policy diffusion**. A health policy can also result chiefly from the spread of innovative practices, rather than from intentional adoption and adaptation of other policies. Such policy diffusion is a sophisticated process in which a strategy (such as management by objective, results-based management or new public management) permeates the public sector and eventually leads to the development of a new health policy (see Box 6, for example).

BOX 6. POLICY DIFFUSION IN GERMANY – AN INDIRECT LINK

In Germany, the translation of Health for All from the international to the national level has taken a roundabout way, and it has been characterized primarily by the spread of innovative thinking about population health. The first attempt to formulate a Health for All policy failed owing to political conditions in the late 1980s and early 1990s. Nevertheless, many German states introduced their own Health for All policies; the first was Hamburg (31,32), which adopted a policy in 1992, followed in 1995 by North Rhine–Westphalia, which chose 10 of the 38 targets in the 1991 European policy update (33).

Germany's second federal attempt to define health targets in 2003 was more successful. However, there was no intentional or systematic effort to adopt Health for All principles, and the WHO policy was considered to be only one among many sources of information and inspiration. For instance, in drafting the federal policy, participants made comparisons of how the different member countries of the Organisation for Economic Co-operation and Development (OECD) had drafted and implemented health targets. They also reviewed various international experiences in setting priorities and formulating an evidence-based health policy.

- **Policy convergence.** Member States can also formulate Health for All policies entirely independently of WHO and its policy frameworks. This path usually occurs in countries with a sustainable tradition that enables them to react independently to common challenges (see Box 7, for example).

BOX 7. POLICY CONVERGENCE IN FRANCE – NO LINK

France provides an example of a Member State initiating a national Health for All policy without reference to the European policy and movement. In 1991, the Haut Comité de la Santé Publique was established by decree under the supervision of the minister responsible for health. The committee's mission has been to improve the health of the population by informing the decision-making process. One of its specific tasks has been to observe population health and help define health policy objectives. It prepared several reports that led to a 1994 general report containing a policy with quantified health targets *(34)*. More reports in 1998 and 2002 contributed to the preparation of a public health bill passed by the French parliament in 2004. The bill primarily seeks to reorganize the disjointed decision-making system in public health; it also contains public health goals and national strategic plans. Some of these documents do indeed refer to the WHO definition of health, and use technical concepts and norms defined and advocated by WHO. But the policy dimension of WHO, particularly the Health for All policy, receives no mention. This was confirmed by interviews conducted with French policy-makers, who recognized that the European Health for All policy had had little influence.

The roles of the European Health for All policy in the formulation of national health policies

The European Health for All policy has played several different roles in Member States' efforts to formulate health policies (see Boxes 8–11, for example). In some cases, the European policy has been a strong

---

BOX 8. LATVIA: INITIATING THE DEVELOPMENT OF A HEALTH POLICY

In the late 1990s, a draft of HEALTH21 was translated and distributed among all the national stakeholders in the Latvian health sector. After public consultations, a special meeting of the Cabinet of Ministers discussed the need for a Latvian Health for All strategy. The government expressed its commitment, and a public health strategy was drafted. This course of events was not unprecedented, however, as another policy inspired by Health for All, entitled "Better living, better Latvia", had been formulated previously.

BOX 9. THE CZECH REPUBLIC: SPARKING DEBATE AND FACILITATING POLICY FORMULATION

In the Czech Republic, the Health for All policy framework triggered debate on formulating a health policy, and for almost 20 years it continued to guide the process. In the 1980s, the country committed itself to implementing a Health for All policy, and the 38 European targets were translated into Czech. Throughout the 1990s, several policies were drafted along Health for All lines, including the Proposal for Reforming the Care of Health (which reflected a multisectoral approach to health promotion) and the National Programme of Health Restoration and Promotion. In 2002, the government approved a long-term strategy for improving the health status of the population, entitled HEALTH21: health for all in the 21st century. The document describes the main goals for national health development, including targets and the means to achieve them.

BOX 10. FINLAND: LEGITIMIZING HEALTH POLICY FORMULATION

The best-documented influence of the European Health for All policy on national policy formulation is found in Finland, where there was a strong push to establish a health policy for which the European policy was instrumental in garnering political support. As early as 1982, just a few years after the Declaration of Alma-Ata and before the launch of the first European Region policy, Finnish institutions were already discussing plans for a comprehensive health policy. With support from the Regional Office, Finland became the first country to test the Region's policy on a national level. From the Finnish perspective, the role of the European policy was to legitimize an already-planned policy and win over its critics.

Having developed a health policy within the Health for All framework back in the 1980s, Poland has just completed its 10-year National Health Programme. The Programme covered the period 1996–2005 and included monitoring of progress in 18 different areas. Evaluation of the Programme shows that Poland achieved population health improvements despite the constraints of a difficult economic transition. Implementation relied strongly on local governments, which launched more than 400 local health programmes. The experience gained is reflected in the new National Health Programme for 2006–2015.

---

instigating factor, setting in motion the development of a national health policy. In other cases, it has facilitated debate during the preparation process. Finally, it has also been used to legitimize a policy that was already planned.

Influencing the subnational level

The spread of Health for All policies to the subnational level should come as no surprise, since subnational entities have political authority, administrative competence and financial responsibility for key public health functions in many European Member States. Despite some common features, though, the formulation of subnational Health for All policies is strongly affected by their particular circumstances, and they show several patterns of emergence (see Box 12).

BOX 12. SUBNATIONAL HEALTH POLICIES

In the United Kingdom, the 1998 devolution acts established separate legislative bodies in Scotland, Wales and Northern Ireland. While the powers granted to each body vary somewhat, health is one of the matters devolved to all three. Decentralization in Spain has also had an impact on health policy development. Though actual activity varies a great deal among the regions, national law obliges each autonomous region to formulate a health policy. In Italy too, the regional health policies are closely linked to the national one. In Germany, half the states have formulated or drafted health policies or health targets. The states have asked the federal government to formulate its own health policy and health targets in order to complement state competencies in health-related areas.

Planning policy funding, infrastructure and monitoring

The Observatory study also surveyed the bridges between policy formulation and implementation. One such bridge is planning the infrastructure and financial resources needed to implement a Health for All policy, as well as the systems needed to monitor it. Planning for these needs inevitably opens up discussion of the potential non-health-related consequences of such a policy. A sustainable policy requires a substantial managerial, medical and scientific infrastructure, as well as sufficient funds to implement and monitor policy measures and interventions. If such things are not planned, it is unlikely that even the best-worded Health for All policy will be implemented successfully.

Of the 40 Health for All policies examined, 32 contain some provision for implementation. Specifically, they address issues of funding, infrastructure and monitoring processes or outcomes.

Have national Health for All policies affected the implementation of health initiatives?

Little or no direct influence

The Observatory study found no evidence that national Health for All policies directly affect health reforms, programmes or projects. While the European Region's Health for All policy has had a strong, often direct influence on the way Member States formulate their national health policies, national Health for All policies have had very little direct influence on the implementation of health activities. Direct WHO involvement appears to have been limited to WHO technical programmes providing advice and assistance of a technical, non-policy nature. Perhaps the study's research methodology and selection of countries contributed to no examples of such influence being found. Recent developments, such as the new French and Swedish health policies, may show greater effects in the near future.

An abundance of soft implementation

The influence of the Health for All concept is felt beyond health policy documents. In some Member States, the national Health for All policy is not the only health policy document, and multiple documents sometimes cross-reference and cross-fertilize each other. Although health reforms, programmes and projects may not derive directly from the Health for All policy, it may still contribute to the consistency of such activities and the context in which they occur (see Box 13).

BOX 13. NORWAY: POLICY DOCUMENTS, PROGRAMMES AND PROJECTS ALIGNED WITH THE NATIONAL HEALTH FOR ALL POLICY (35)

- Smoking ban in bars, restaurants etc. (from 1 June 2004)
- Action plan to prevent unwanted pregnancies and abortions (2004–2008)
- "Together for mental health in Norway" – the government's strategic plan for the mental health of children and young people
- Escalation plan for mental health
- Reform to provide patients with a choice of regular general practitioner
- Municipal care services
- Hospital reform
- Right to choose hospitals programme
- New act on alternative treatments of disease

National Health for All policies can indeed support policy implementation, but such support is usually diffuse and not directly associated with a particular programme or project. A national Health for All policy may do any of the following things.

- **Change national perceptions on certain issues**. This effect has been reported in Finland, despite its long track record in health policy formulation and implementation and its status as the first European country to develop a Health for All policy. Changing perceptions can be an important first step in influencing decision-making and implementing new programmes and projects.

- **Influence the decision-making process**. Again in Finland, public health advocates found it effective to refer to the European policy framework, since it had been devised by a respected international organization and endorsed by its Member States.

- **Provide a common orientation for public health activists, health professionals and members of the academic public health community**. This important if indirect type of influence proved valuable in the United Kingdom when health equity issues were not on the national political agenda. The national Health for All policy provided a framework for local health policy development and implementation in England. In Sweden, a national initiative to address all the key determinants of population health is being used to refocus health policy and ways of working across sectors.

- **Help justify improvements in health system infrastructure**. In Kazakhstan, the national policy was an instrumental factor in establishing the Kazakhstan School of Public Health.

Independent implementation of individual elements

When a Health for All policy is in place, some of its concepts may be successfully implemented, even though the policy itself has not influenced their implementation. While it may sound paradoxical, several cases illustrate such uncoupled implementation. For instance, sometimes a programme, project or piece of legislation is implemented prior to the relevant policy formulation.

5. Ethical governance and the Health for All values

Introduction

Shared values

Across the European Region, certain common values play a central role in health decision-making. It is true that there are large variations among and within European societies, and that the health and social sector of the modern European welfare state is constantly changing. Nevertheless, these shared core values extend beyond health and permeate all sectors of society. Together they comprise a social consensus – a sense of collective social purpose and a belief in fairness – that creates a solid foundation for fair, socially responsible government. These values include a commitment to the social good, solidarity, universal participation and a belief in the need for strict public regulation *(36,37)*.

There is scarcely any country in the WHO European Region where it would be acceptable or expedient for a national health authority to declare that it did not stand for justice, equity, solidarity or widespread participation, or to take actions that imperilled these values. Nor does any European society conceive of health and health care services as standard market commodities that can be privatized for profit (see Box 14). These widespread beliefs in what is and is not acceptable have framed national health sector debate and promoted strong international bonds within the Region. Naturally, each country makes its own choice of how to put these values into practice. In general, even profit-making providers of health care services are

---

BOX 14. HEALTH CARE FOR SALE?

Rather than regarding most curative and preventive health care services as ordinary market commodities, Europeans understand them to be a social good, believing that universal provision of such services will benefit society through a higher standard of living and greater social cohesion. In Spain, for example, Article 43 of the 1978 Constitution recognizes the right to health protection and requires public authorities to organize and oversee public health activities, including preventive measures. And the Cohesion and Quality in the National Health System Act, which was recently passed, requires the coordination of public health care bodies in order to guarantee citizens their right to health protection. Both legal instruments aim to ensure equity and quality in the Spanish health care system.

---

sensitive to the national ethical context. This is especially true with regard to the functioning of health systems, owing to the increasing tendency to blur at times the boundaries between public and private in the health sector, e.g. to involve the private sector in public health activities.

One major challenge in putting these shared values into practice is to ensure sound financing of health systems so that they can function in a way that respects Health for All. In many countries, policy-makers face the need to pool resources in a way that is socially fair with respect to wealth, so that those who have more will lend support to those who have less.

The values in their political context

The ways in which values permeate health policy-making are complex, for several reasons.

Reaching a common understanding of broad ethical notions can be a complicated task, especially in a Europe that is changing rapidly. Values are subject to interpretation, and there are no common definitions that Member States and health stakeholders would all acknowledge to be both standard and precise. Throughout the European Region, there are numerous examples of the same word (including "equity" and "solidarity") having several distinct meanings. This situation causes difficulties when values must be applied in specific settings. One way to deal with it is to analyse values in a human rights framework, an approach that can help policy-makers establish baseline values that are fundamental, immutable and widely held.

At times, respect for values can pull policy-makers in conflicting directions. Ethical governance involves continually grappling with necessary trade-offs – for example, between equity and cost–effectiveness. Policy-makers have to make tough choices about which values to uphold and prioritize, and how much compromise is acceptable, in so far as values are only one among many factors that influence policy-making.

Values sometimes remain peripheral because of difficulty in determining how they affect the actual implementation of policies. While declarations of the importance of values often appear in the preambles to national health policy documents, translating them from rhetoric into a basis for action is another matter. Values may be interesting but they can also seem abstract and impractical, and it is difficult to verify, monitor and measure their implementation.

The way forward

It is hoped that this update's re-examination of Health for All values will render them more useful and relevant and thus encourage their practical implementation. The values appear to be endorsed by the Region's Member States and, as indicated in Chapter 4, a large number of governments have referred to them explicitly in formulating their national health policies. Yet declaring the significance of these values does not mean that they are necessarily driving health systems, and several important questions still need to be raised.

- What role do values play in the Region's national health sectors?
- Which values are valid for the European health sector in the 21st century?
- Do these values also lie at the heart of policies formulated in other sectors – particularly the major policies dealing with national social and economic development?
- How can these values be understood better, and how can they be made more useful to policy-makers?

- What kinds of mechanisms would contribute to the practical implementation of these values?

To address these questions, the present update offers two possible approaches – two frameworks for working with health policy values.

- **Legal**. Values form the basis for the legal human rights framework, which includes the international obligations that countries have incurred in negotiating and approving various human rights instruments. Europe is relatively advanced in this area, with strong regional instruments to which its countries have committed themselves.

- **Ethical**. Values also play a major part in the shared ethical framework of moral norms and standards of conduct that are accepted by all countries and generally respected by all the actors in each. Decisions and actions can thus be measured against this framework.

Instead of favouring either framework over the other, there are several good reasons to combine them. The two frameworks are complementary rather than mutually exclusive; both are susceptible to progressive realization, negotiation, interpretation and adjustment; and neither should trump the other, or be more important or influential, in modern societies.

Considering values within both frameworks simultaneously can assist policy-makers in developing ethical, values-based governance. This approach assumes that a health system can be evaluated at any level with respect to both commonly agreed ethical norms and legally binding human rights norms. Values may thus be used to test, evaluate and improve the performance of a health system, just as they can be used to evaluate governance in general. Such assessment is most useful if carried out by the individual country. In considering the Region's social consensus, a country may also wish to reassert its own commitment to it. Adhering to such basic, commonly shared values has become especially useful today, when national policy-makers often receive conflicting views about the most effective way to strengthen their health systems.

Combining the legal and ethical approaches also offers some pragmatic ways to understand and implement the Health for All values. While primarily useful to policy-makers, this joint approach can also be useful for a range of other stakeholders in the sector – nongovernmental organizations, the population at large, professional organizations, political parties, the academic and research subsector and even private firms.

Health in the legal human rights framework

The right to health

As mentioned before, the WHO Constitution states that, "The enjoyment of the highest attainable standard of health is one of the fundamental rights of every human being". This vision guides the work of WHO with its Member States. For the individual, the right to health does not mean the right to be healthy; rather, it is a claim for a set of social arrangements, norms and laws that can provide everyone with the opportunity to reach his or her full health potential. For a government, the right to health implies it has a responsibility to ensure that everyone in its jurisdiction can realize this right as fully as possible. This responsibility may be fulfilled through numerous complementary approaches, such as the formulation of health policies, the implementation of health programmes and the adoption of specific legal instruments. Governments are not only obliged to work toward positive health outcomes; they also have to ensure that health facilities, goods and services are broadly available, accessible, affordable and of high quality, particularly with respect to the most vulnerable and marginalized population groups (23,38). Finally, the right to health implies a right not only to health care but also to disease prevention, health protection and health promotion.

In a national context, the right to health is often pragmatically regarded as the right to certain entitlements – the specific health services that a country's laws guarantee its inhabitants.

The broad context of human rights

Although the right to health can be considered the flagship right in the formulation of health policy, the human rights approach to health also draws on other human rights, norms and principles. Most of them are described in the Universal Declaration of Human Rights – the founding document of the human rights movement and a declaration that has been almost universally endorsed. Applying the human rights approach to the practical world of health systems is relatively new to both the health and human rights sectors, and it means acknowledging some general rights that do not refer explicitly to health:

- the right to equal treatment and freedom from discrimination;
- the right to free, meaningful and effective participation;
- the right to seek and receive information;
- the right to benefit from scientific progress and its applications;
- the right to a healthy physical and social environment;
- the right to clean water, safe food and adequate housing; and
- the right to privacy.

The human rights approach is particularly relevant for the health sector because considering each of these rights has direct consequences for the design, monitoring, implementation and evaluation of national health policies and programmes *(39)*.

Health and human rights are closely interrelated. Health is affected by many social, economic, environmental, cultural and political factors and, as noted above, respecting the right to health requires that other human rights be respected, too. The relationship may be described as threefold.

First, direct violations of human rights can have a clear and often severe impact on the health of the persons affected. Second, the way in which some public health policies and programmes are designed or implemented may result in indirect violations of human rights. Third, directly or indirectly, health is a prerequisite for most other human rights that have been recognized in international treaties. When health has been impaired, it can be difficult for individuals to exercise their right to act as full members of their communities.

Every Member State in the WHO European Region has signed at least one treaty, convention or other international instrument that commits it to respecting human rights.

It is difficult for any country to guarantee immediately and completely the rights addressed by such instruments, because doing so requires not only passing appropriate laws but also implementing a number of administrative, financial, educational and social measures. That is why it is widely recognized that the achievement of human rights requires "progressive realization", which is understood as making continual progress on human rights as expeditiously as possible. This approach is extremely relevant to health policy too, although many of the professionals involved in developing health systems and policies may not be sufficiently aware of its advantages.

Referring to the international commitments undertaken by their respective states confers several substantial benefits for health ministries.

- Such international obligations buttress health policy-making values with legal entitlements and international standards.

- Health policy-makers are better equipped than anyone else to help the rest of the government understand how their country's international commitments relate to health.

- When ratifying international treaties, countries often devise and agree to national human rights benchmarks against which progress is to be measured. Health policy-makers can adopt and use these benchmarks.

- The fundamental rights and values enshrined in international instruments and national legislation contain important guidance on structuring and improving a country's health system and dealing respectfully with members of the public.

- The human rights approach can help governments avoid discrimination, especially against members of vulnerable and marginalized groups, due to inadequately targeted health policies and programmes.

- Like other human rights, the right to health does not belong to any particular group. More specifically, it belongs not just to patients but to a population as a whole.

Health in the shared ethical framework: the Health for All values

In the shared ethical framework, there is no ultimate, one-size-fits-all, now-and-forever answer to which values are important. During a particular period, certain values may become widely accepted as fundamental in a given country. However, such agreement is unlikely to apply everywhere. Throughout the European Region, there are many examples of communication failures that occurred when different actors used the same words to mean completely different things. In a geographic area that is changing so rapidly – especially one that is home to dozens of different languages – it is difficult to achieve agreement on broadly conceived ethical notions. That is why this update calls for values to be referred to in their specific contexts. For health policy-makers, this is in itself an ethical choice – to grapple with the difficulties of implementing values by forgoing the political comfort of using them only as rhetorical flourishes, and instead, looking honestly at how values relate to the practical exigencies of devising and implementing policies.

In accordance with both the vision articulated in this update and the best recent thinking in health policy studies, three basic values have been identified as essential Health for All values: equity, solidarity and participation. National health decision-makers have numerous opportunities to decide precisely how to put these values into practice. While every national health policy reflects a national agenda in the way it addresses health needs and political and economic realities, if it is a true Health for All policy, it cannot ignore these three core values.

Equity

In the Health for All context, equity implies that everyone has a fair opportunity to attain their full health potential, and that no one is prevented from achieving this potential if at all possible. Based on this definition, a health policy based on equity would seek to eliminate or minimize avoidable differences in health outcomes: it would promote equity of opportunity in achieving one's full health potential. It would ensure that health treatments are available to all, regardless of such factors as patient gender, age, social condition, financial resources, ethnicity, religious belief, sexual orientation, national origin, educational level, geographic location, political opinions and citizenship status. Equity concerns also extend to numerous aspects of the provision and distribution of health services, health gains, health resources and health information. As mentioned previously, such services encompass not just health care but also prevention, health promotion and public health efforts.

In the public health sector, equity may be understood in two ways.

- **Equity in process** means the government has made sure that all people have an equal opportunity to access health services that are tailored to their individual needs, independent of their ability to contribute to the system.

- **Equity in outcome** means the government has done everything it can to bring the potential for health that members of disadvantaged groups have up to the level that the rest of the population enjoys. Outcome equity can be increased by, for example, instituting specific compensatory mechanisms for social groups that are underprivileged owing to various vulnerabilities, so long as such mechanisms are acceptable to these groups.

It is essential to interpret and implement equity in the context of health systems. In pursuing the fundamental goal of health gains, equity means to reduce unfair differences in health status among individuals, social groups, regions etc.

Equity and human rights
Equity is closely linked to human rights. In considering equity in the legal human rights framework, the importance of providing equal opportunities for health becomes evident. Inequity in health status

refers to differences that are not only systematic and quantifiable but avoidable as well. Inequity thus refers to differences that are unfair and avoidable. Equity is a normative ethical value that entails fair distribution of resources and access within and among various population groups.

In the health field, equity efforts include reducing any discrimination in access to the benefits of health initiatives. A comprehensive programme to promote equity requires striking the right balance between two perspectives – the consideration of health determinants and of health needs. From the viewpoint of health determinants, an equity programme should seek to minimize the effect of all underlying health determinants that create unequal opportunities for people with similar needs. This is known as horizontal equity. From the viewpoint of health needs, an equity programme should focus on people with greater medical needs – vertical equity (40,41). Thus, as stated in Article 2 of the Universal Declaration of Human Rights (42), equity reinforces every person's entitlement to the enjoyment of human rights and freedoms "without distinction of any kind".

Sometimes the pursuit of equity leads to the application of different standards to different groups in order to compensate for existing inequalities. (This practice is sometimes called "positive discrimination", a term that should be used with caution owing to connotations that are in fact negative.) Equity efforts may therefore be seen as compensatory mechanisms that decrease certain existing disparities in health between more and less advantaged population groups, within and between countries.

Equity in health policy
In order to assess the extent to which equity in health has been achieved, policy-makers need to consider assorted socioeconomic, cultural and environmental factors. As indicated above, this requires examining the broader context of all potential health determinants that might situate people at different social levels and thus disadvantage some groups. A prime example of a health determinant to consider is poverty in its various manifestations – an uncertain food supply, social exclusion and discrimination, inadequate housing, insufficient protection of early

childhood development and unsafe labour conditions, not to mention poor quality health services. Poverty accounts for most of the global burden of disease and death, and for the bulk of existing health inequities between and within countries. These effects are socially determined and can be best addressed through specific poverty reduction strategies and health policies that confront poverty as a cause of ill health.

To obtain insight into the complex causes of health disparities, policy-makers can institute mechanisms to register and evaluate the degree of health inequities among different social groups, as well as the extent to which health policies and programmes have been successful in improving the health of vulnerable and disadvantaged groups.

In the health sector, equity should be a concern not only in health care but also in the realms of prevention, health promotion and public health. This point is essential in evaluating which health services should be covered by public funds and how the overall health services budget should be allocated. To this end, a policy that promotes equity should not be satisfied with focusing on individual lifestyles or the needs of marginalized and vulnerable groups. The vast majority of the population is affected negatively by at least one health determinant, and the existing inequalities in health call for health policies to address all social and economic health determinants.

However, health equity cannot be seen as the responsibility of the health sector alone; it needs to be treated as an intersectoral issue. Social parameters such as income, housing or education have a great effect on health status, and health equity depends substantially on the implementation of appropriate policies in all public sectors. As a consequence, health sector policies and programmes that seek to improve the health of all citizens should consider collaborating with any relevant actor, whether inside or outside the government, and whether concerned primarily with social, educational, environmental or legislative issues.

Solidarity
Solidarity is usually defined as a society's sense of collective responsibility. In the health sector, solidarity means that everyone contributes to the

health system according to ability to pay, rather than utilization of health services. Solidarity is thus about the distribution of resources: who pays how much, for what and when. The distribution of health gains is still not equal in even the richest countries, and solidarity ensures that the funding burden is distributed fairly and equitably. In this respect, solidarity means reduction of the direct interdependence between what an individual pays and the services received. In a Health for All system, commitment to solidarity is critical, as it means that the system makes health services available to everybody, even citizens who have limited financial resources. Solidarity is the value ensuring that the funding burden is distributed in a fair and equitable way. Fair processes are increasingly recognized as a necessity for various institutions at different levels of decision-making *(43)*.

Solidarity and individual responsibility
Many European societies recognize that people are partly responsible for their own health. Because there are limits to attainable health, there are limits to solidarity, too. A typical example is the debate on whether interventions regarded as "luxurious" or "extra" should be covered by public funds. The answers vary from country to country, and even among countries firmly committed to solidarity, such coverage varies greatly. Indeed, decisions about the essential content of solidarity-based health care services are essentially political decisions, ordinarily taking into account not only needs assessments but also resource availability. Sometimes, a country committed to solidarity will exclude from its list of routine services treatments and preventive measures that may be cost-effective in a specific case or setting but not cost-effective on a large scale. Thus, determining the benefits package is a process grounded in the ethical norms of the society at large. It does not lessen the central role of individuals in protecting their own health, through healthy lifestyles, compliance with medical advice etc. (see Box 15).

The interrelatedness of solidarity and equity
The distinction in health systems between solidarity and equity can be artificial at times. Solidarity is one of the means to achieve equity. Equity implies that the state has instituted compensatory mechanisms so that all population groups receive services according to need.

In Slovenia, cervical cancer screening was introduced to regular gynaecological practice in 1960. Nonetheless, since 1994 the country has seen an upward trend in the national incidence of the disease, and in 2000, it was one of the highest in Europe. One of the reasons was that only 30% of Slovene women were being screened, despite all of them having nominally equal access to the procedure. Especially when participation was left to individual initiative, the screening system frequently missed older women and women from lower socioeconomic groups, even though both groups were at higher risk for the disease.

A pilot project to tackle the problem was established in 1998. Through a link to the Central Population Register of Slovenia, cervical cancer screenings were monitored, and personal invitations were sent to all women in the target age group of 20 to 64 years. It resulted in nearly a 50% participation rate among those women who had not been regularly screened before. In 2003, the National Programme of Organized Cervical Cancer Screening was launched. It advocates active population-wide prevention measures based on scientific methods and quality control procedures. By having Slovenia's compulsory health insurance fund cover participation, the health system has ensured universal access to the programme, thereby demonstrating its commitment to equity and solidarity.

Measures introduced to increase solidarity can lead to similar results. Both core values can also be assessed by evaluating how even-handed the system is – by determining whether the society as a whole gauges government health policies, decisions and actions to be fair.

In this respect, fairness means that the poor should not pay more than the rich as a percentage of their disposable income: people contribute to a solidarity-based system in proportion to their ability to pay. Such fairness in financial contributions is one of the core goals of Health for All systems, and yet another example of how fundamentally values permeate the functioning of health systems. This concept is especially relevant to economic transition countries that are carrying out major health reforms. In such cases, it is always tempting to compromise equity and solidarity for the immediate prospect of achieving maximum cost–effectiveness and reaping the highest possible health gains from very limited financial resources – a temptation that is one of the greatest challenges to ethical, values-based governance. In systems with multiple health insurers, maintaining solidarity in health care requires strict regulation and explicit guidelines in order to prevent them from violating the principle of equity by competing for healthier, lower-risk groups.

Solidarity as a driving force behind participation

A society that practises solidarity requires everyone's participation. When solidarity is enshrined in the law, it often indicates the involvement of people who have sought to elevate their sense of social justice to law. In this respect, public accountability is essential – in a society that respects solidarity, health authorities should be held accountable for its implementation and for demonstrating whether and how solidarity brings the desired social benefits.

Participation

For the purposes of this update, participation is defined as the direct involvement of people, either individually or collectively, to influence health decision-making in the public sector.

Providing information to the general public and consulting them about their views are the two most basic forms of public participation. Member States in the European Region have developed increasingly innovative ways of involving the public in areas such as setting health priorities and ascertaining levels of satisfaction with health services.

Another form of collective public participation occurs through patient and consumer advocacy groups. European countries have seen marked growth in these groups, and they appear to contribute to the public policy debate of pluralistic societies positively and effectively. In some instances, however, a group advocates the special interests of particular clients or disease groups that do not reflect broader societal health needs and interests (see Box 16).

Increased patient participation in health care decisions

Patients are being increasingly involved in their treatment decisions, but the trend is a complex one. It is essential to balance patient involvement with professional medical opinion. On the one hand, informing patients about their cases and involving them in clinical decisions has proven to be beneficial, especially when there is some uncertainty in diagnosis

---

BOX 16. PARTICIPATION IN LATVIA

A negative case
Many groups in Latvia seek to organize, support and educate patients and to influence health care decision-making. Doctors often participate in such organizations and serve in leadership roles. However, pharmaceutical companies are frequently the main sponsors of such associations, sometimes for less than philanthropic reasons. For instance, a Latvian menopause association has been actively promoting hormone replacement therapy while remaining silent about the fact that this therapy is no longer widely accepted by the international research community. The association thus appears to be advancing the interests of a pharmaceutical company rather than those of the patient community it purports to represent.

A positive case
The Patients' Rights Office of Latvia was established by lawyers. They refer to themselves as a nongovernmental organization made up of patient representatives, since they are not themselves patients but a professional, neutral party that represents patients with no stake of its own. The Office seeks to promote a better national understanding of international human rights and patients' rights instruments, and it has positively influenced health care decision-making, legislative efforts and mass media coverage.

---

or prognosis, or when there are trade-offs among alternative courses of action. In such cases, a patient's values, expectations and priorities should play a central role in making treatment decisions. On the other hand, health professionals continue to bear the responsibility for choosing the best form of treatment, and professional opinions ought to carry special weight. Still, assigning responsibility to a professional should not exclude patient participation or be regarded as elevating the professional over the patient. Clearly presented professional input actually facilitates patient participation. In addition, the expression of patient viewpoints and experiences is useful not only in clinical care but also in health policy-making.

Greater consumer choice: benefits and risks

Increasingly, countries in the European Region give patients free choice of primary care providers and hospital providers. Many Europeans regard patient choice as the best way for people to influence health services effectively. While as a participatory mechanism it can indeed influence policy and help create more responsive health systems, patient choice can also incur additional costs. Moreover, it may undermine solidarity and increase health inequities. There is ample evidence showing that the higher and better-informed social classes tend to benefit most from patient choice, while for vulnerable or more disadvantaged groups it makes little difference.

The policy challenge

Even participatory mechanisms that have been instituted with good intentions sometimes ignore the needs of vulnerable groups, such as people who are mentally disabled, migrant, elderly and alone, or HIV-positive. It is crucial for health policy-makers to acknowledge the interests of special groups such as these, and not to respond to concerns about the negative effects of participatory mechanisms by simply cutting back on them (by decreasing choice). Instead, policy-makers should focus their efforts on increasing access to information. In particular, they should actively support the participation of the most underprivileged and vulnerable groups, whose members tend to lack experience and confidence in making their voices heard. Possible means include incorporating the promotion of participation and patients' rights into policies and legal instruments. Another such opportunity lies in regional policies that have already been adopted by individual Member States: for instance, citizens have the right to public participation and information on the state of their environment.

One sign that public participation is becoming truly effective is that health decision-makers are being held accountable for their decisions. Mechanisms that enforce and ensure accountability include:

- formal consumer representation on management boards, such as those of insurers, health authorities and hospital providers;
- enumeration of the rights and responsibilities of both health providers and citizens;
- the institution of complaint procedures; and
- the increased involvement of health personnel in assessing the actual benefits of health policies and in monitoring their effects on access, acceptability and quality of care, especially for members of disadvantaged and vulnerable groups.

Ethical, values-based governance

In the European welfare state, the government is traditionally responsible for ensuring that health systems are ethically developed and managed. The present update interprets this as a call for health policy-makers to ensure that:

- fundamental human rights are respected in their country; and
- the values of equity, solidarity and participation are prominent, supported and implemented.

The way to link these values to actual action is ethical governance.

Of course, the practice of governance varies widely from one country to another. Moreover, the degree to which it is ethical is often influenced by factors that lie outside the health system, such as peace and social and political stability, as well as the presence (and nature) of vested interests, financial resources and leadership. To further complicate the situation, many European health systems have recently undergone radical transformations.

Ethical governance in the health sectors of the European Region is a natural outgrowth of the European Health for All movement. It can manifest itself in several ways: evidence-based decision-making, primacy of primary health care, multisectoral cooperation or a special emphasis on the needs of disadvantaged groups. Accountability and transparency should in any case be indispensable, since ethical governance should establish mechanisms to enhance these values at every level. Accountability and transparency also make it easier to assess how well national health policies, programmes and initiatives conform to national values.

The value of values

A strong ethical foundation can be invaluable in trying to improve system performance, and experiences from several of the Region's Member States suggest that, during periods of health system reform, loyalty to core Health for All values is a worthwhile goal. In some countries, ethical performance is now regarded as a key element of overall health system performance, along with clinical and financial performance. This development represents a shift towards a recognition of values as an increasingly important constituent in the practical implementation of health policy, since improving system performance requires a combination of vision, technical knowledge and the ability to manage change. In other words, ethical, values-based governance can help provide the necessary vision and foundation for changes that will improve health system performance.

Ethical governance in health means that both the legal human rights framework and the shared ethical framework are brought to the foreground in making decisions and in developing and evaluating health policies, programmes and initiatives. To do so effectively, national health policy-makers may find it useful to have tools to help them assess whether, and to what extent, the decisions they make are in accordance with the core Health for All values (see Chapter 6).

Finally, since an ethical approach is especially important to the effective stewardship and governance function of health systems, it should inform every policy or action that may affect population health, regardless of the sector it originates in. A nation's health sector needs to work together with other public sectors, and this coordination has its ethical dimension. In Europe, policy-makers from non-health sectors would hardly question the importance of solidarity and equity to a health initiative. They should be likewise urged to evaluate any decision that lies in their domain not only for its potential health repercussions but also for its reinforcement of Health for All values.

6. A Health for All toolbox: practical ways to implement the Health for All values

This chapter describes a variety of instruments, actions, methods and techniques, some well established and others still being developed. Health ministries can use these handy tools in designing and implementing policies that promote health for all. They can help policy-makers look at traditional public health areas from new perspectives, map out the values they want to drive their policies, and uphold these values in practice. The toolbox contains policy documents, treaties, agencies and institutions, networks, practices and concepts, methodologies, databases and initiatives.

None of the tools and methods described below was developed specifically to implement the Health for All values. Most of them have already proven useful at the country level and are now being used by policy-makers. Depending on circumstances, these tools can be used as they are, adapted to specific conditions and needs, or serve as inspiration for developing additional approaches.

Rather than attempting to give a comprehensive list of all such tools, this chapter presents 10 that exemplify the range of what is available to policy-makers who want to work towards the goal of health for all.

To facilitate use, the 10 examples have been arranged in four groups, corresponding to four basic questions about how to proceed.

- How can health policy-makers establish a framework for ethical governance?

- How can they incorporate up-to-date data into their health policies?
- How can they assess the implementation of policy values?
- How can they further rationalize health policies and actions?

How can health policy-makers establish a framework for ethical governance?

TOOL ONE – Turn obligations into opportunities: international human rights instruments

International treaties and covenants contain legally binding obligations for the governments of signatory nations – an essential tool in the hands of health ministries. A country is obliged to amend its national legislation as necessary to fulfil these commitments, and health officials who are familiar with them can refer to them proactively. They can use these international instruments to assess existing policies, to propose changes and to engage other actors in the sector in active debate. Decision-makers, lawmakers and nongovernmental organizations can also use them to make health-related changes in areas such as finance, justice and education.

The global perspective: United Nations treaties
The Universal Declaration of Human Rights is the framework for all international human rights law. According to Article 25, "Everyone has the right to a standard of living adequate for the health and well-being of himself and his family, including food, clothing, housing and medical care and necessary social services". This article forms the basis for the entire construction of the right to health. The right to health is further specified in seven major United Nations covenants and conventions, which also have legal force (see Box 17). Each agreement contains at least one article that directly concerns the right to health, as well as other articles that indirectly address health and the conditions for health.

The implementation of these foundational human rights treaties is monitored by committees of independent experts ("treaty monitoring bodies"), created under the auspices of and supported by the United

> ### BOX 17. UNITED NATIONS HUMAN RIGHTS TREATIES
>
> The International Covenant on Economic, Social and Cultural Rights (ICESCR) provides the most authoritative interpretation of the right to health. A General Comment on the right to health clarifies the nature of relevant individual rights and state obligations *(21)*. The General Comment defines the right to health as an inclusive right, embracing the right not only to timely and appropriate health care but also to the underlying determinants of health, including adequate water quality, housing, food, environmental quality, living and working conditions and information. It also says that the right to health is not to be understood as the right to be healthy, but rather as encompassing certain freedoms (control over one's body, sexual and reproductive rights, and freedom from torture and medical experimentation) and entitlements (to a system of health protection). Finally, it states that the state should ensure the population's participation in all health-related decision-making at every level of government.

Nations. States that are party to a treaty are required to submit regular reports on how they are meeting their treaty obligations. Under some of the conventions, individuals and organizations may also register complaints of rights violations.

Other major United Nations human rights instruments include the International Covenant on Civil and Political Rights (ICCPR), the International Convention on the Elimination of All Forms of Racial Discrimination (ICERD), the Convention on the Elimination of All Forms of Discrimination against Women (CEDAW), the Convention on the Rights of the Child (CRC), the Convention against Torture and Other Cruel, Inhuman or Degrading Treatment or Punishment (CAT) and the International Convention on the Protection of the Rights of All Migrant Workers and Members of Their Families (CMW).

The European perspective

The Council of Europe human rights system
Convention for the Protection of Human Rights and Fundamental Freedoms, also known as the European Convention on Human Rights, or ECHR *(44)*. A major postulate of this convention is that the right to health derives from the right to life. It also addresses a number of related rights: the right to human dignity, the right to the protection of privacy and personal data, and the right to private and

family life. Parties to the ECHR undertake to secure all these rights and freedoms to everyone in their jurisdictions. The ECHR has also established international enforcement mechanisms.

European Court of Human Rights (Strasbourg). The Court hears petitions from individuals, groups and states regarding violations of the ECHR by parties to it. In pronouncing upon specific cases, the Court sometimes elaborates on the explicit content of the right to health. For instance, it has stated that the right to health implies a state's obligation to protect its inhabitants against unnecessary risks to their health by implementing preventive measures, instituting effective mechanisms, guaranteeing an appropriate balance of individual and collective rights and avoiding any degrading or inhuman treatment.

European Social Charter. The rights that the Charter guarantees to all individuals involve provisions for accessible and effective health care facilities, prevention policies, the elimination of occupational hazards and the protection of maternity *(45)*.

European Committee of Social Rights. This body determines whether or not national law and practice in Council of Europe Member States are in conformity with their commitments to the European Social Charter. Each state that is party to the Charter must submit an annual report on its legislative and administrative implementation of the Charter.

The European Union (EU) system
Treaty of Amsterdam. Article 152 stipulates that "a high level of human health protection shall be ensured in the definition and implementation of all Community policies and activities" *(46)*.

Charter of Fundamental Rights of the European Union. While it lacks legal force, the Charter is an important statement by the EU Member States, in so far as it gathers in a single document all the civil, political and social rights that are granted to EU citizens *(47)*. Chapter 4, on solidarity, sets out the right to social security and assistance, and to protection in case of maternity, illness, workplace accident or old age; the right to access preventive health care; and the right to receive medical treatment.

Court of Justice of the European Communities. The Court can be brought into health-related cases on various grounds, and it delivers judgment with reference to the international or European instruments that EU Member States have adopted. The Court bases its rulings on the principles set out in the ECHR. Other important agreements that the court refers to include the International Labour Organization (ILO) conventions, the European Social Charter and the International Covenant on Civil and Political Rights (ICCPR).

The effectiveness and limits of international instruments
The most commonly recognized weakness of international instruments is their lack of sanctioning mechanisms. Within the United Nations system of treaty monitoring, there does exist a system of country reports, which provide broad opportunities to publicize and debate basic human rights issues. Country reports to the United Nations can serve as important catalysts for such debates. Ultimately, however, the monitoring bodies have no recourse when a country is passive or hesitates to implement necessary changes, nor can they oblige a country to share reports with the general public. As for Court of Justice decisions, they have proven to have a significant long-term (if somewhat dilatory) impact – in most cases, they are eventually incorporated into national legislation.

There also exist, in certain technical areas such as tobacco control and the environment, other international legal instruments that can be used in a similar manner.

TOOL TWO – Set international goals: the Millennium Development Goals (MDGs)
In 2000, representatives from 189 countries adopted the United Nations Millennium Declaration. It declares that certain principles and values are fundamental for international relations in the 21st century and identifies eight development goals that every country is to strive to meet by 2015. Goals 4, 5 and 6 are directly health-related, addressing child mortality, maternal health, and HIV and other diseases, respectively. After the Declaration was adopted, the United Nations Development Programme (UNDP), the International Monetary Fund (IMF) and the

OECD helped develop 18 precise targets and 48 quantified assessment indicators for the eight goals.

Progress towards the MDGs is monitored via country reports that analyse changes in the indicators. The indicators are designed to measure, target by target, each population's health improvement or decline – thus acting as a mechanism that promotes fairness and solidarity, and making it possible to compare the success of the various states and regions in accomplishing their goals. However, the indicators themselves are still technically imperfect, and policy-makers need to recognize two of their major limitations:

- the quality of information varies from country to country; and
- the indicators reflect only national averages, without providing information on disadvantaged groups or other subpopulations that the targets are especially concerned with.

In the European Region, it is widely recognized that the MDG indicators give only approximate figures and can hide certain inequities. Likewise, the national data being gathered are often inadequate, notably for the goals targeting poverty, child mortality and maternal health.

The link to Health for All values

The emphasis in the MDGs on equity, particularly through global and regional poverty reduction, is consonant with the Health for All vision. Recent EU efforts to reduce poverty through debt relief, new financing mechanisms, and increased development aid provide a good example of how the international community is making an intensified effort to achieve the MDGs.

Other MDGs also relate directly to national Health for All efforts. They include Goal 7, "Ensure environmental sustainability", since water supply, water quality and sanitation are still a problematic health determinant for some countries and subpopulations, and Goal 8, "Develop global partnerships for development", since its call to address development work in a holistic and sustainable manner corresponds to the Health for All call for a broad vision of health partnerships that reach beyond the health sector.

A full examination of the links between health and development requires further delving into the links between equity and development (see Box 18), and WHO is planning to explore these connections in its 2006 world health report.

BOX 18. EUROPEAN OFFICE FOR INVESTMENT FOR HEALTH AND DEVELOPMENT

In January 2000, WHO established the Commission on Macroeconomics and Health to put health on the world economic development agenda. Subsequently, the WHO Regional Office for Europe opened the European Office for Investment for Health and Development in Venice to better understand and act on health determinants in the European Region. The Venice office is charged with analysing the specific situation of each low-income country in the Region and designing health actions adapted to its particular circumstances. One of the Venice office's research projects, a European adaptation of the Commission on Macroeconomics and Health report, analyses the relevance of the MDGs in a European context. Another project focuses on official development assistance for health to the countries of eastern Europe and central Asia. It provides clear evidence that the level of such assistance for health that has been targeted for this part of the Region is far too low compared to need.

TOOL THREE – Enforce public participation

Using the views and expectations of the general public in developing health policy is a relatively recent practice. Its benefits are set forth strongly in the Amsterdam Declaration on the Promotion of Patients' Rights in Europe, and in the Ljubljana Charter on Reforming Health Care. According to these documents, public involvement and empowerment are the best way to design a health system that reflects the needs, values and preferences of the population, while encouraging it at the same time to embrace healthy behaviours. The Council of Europe's Committee of Ministers has also recommended that governments grant their citizens a central role in making decisions that concern their own health, based on what it calls their fundamental right to define the goals of health policy.

It is up to each Member State in the European Region to design appropriate policies to encourage participation (see Boxes 19 and 20). Having gradually recognized the need for such involvement, several western European countries have experimented with various ways to address it, most notably through open public debates. An

---

BOX 19. CONSENSUS CONFERENCES

This method was developed during the 1970s in the United States of America and Canada, mainly as a professional tool to establish medical guidelines. The United Kingdom and France later experimented with consensus conferences during the 1990s, and Denmark has used them as a fundamental option in policy development. A consensus conference involves a panel whose members represent either a population group with a particular health condition or the public at large. Members receive prior information on the issue to be discussed, and they then attend an ad hoc meeting where they listen to experts explaining the potentially controversial aspects. Commentaries and auditions follow, and the panel, which acts as a jury, makes its recommendations. The recommendations usually receive wide media coverage and stimulate public debate, and the decision-makers then consider them for possible incorporation in regulatory decisions. This method has proven successful in encouraging broad public involvement in formulating policies that respect Health for All values.

BOX 20. NATIONAL HEALTH FORUMS

A national health forum is an exchange of views on a topic for which public opinion is considered critical. The preparatory period can last months and may have different formats (workshops, plenary sessions, private work groups). Public forums usually receive a lot of press coverage, which stimulates further debate. They provide a space where personal experience, professional (and sometimes corporate) opinions, and various kinds of data (technical, financial and scientific) can meet. In France, the Etats Généraux de la Santé enjoyed broad participation, with national and regional conferences taking place on a regular basis. The process led to a 2004 law defining the roles of patients and their representative organizations in health care systems. In the United Kingdom, the Department of Health launched a large national consultation in 2004. The white paper *Choosing health* posed wide-ranging questions on how the country might tackle preventable problems such as obesity, smoking and sexually transmitted infections. This document formed the basis for a nationwide consultation exercise, with hundreds of events across the country organized by national and local authorities and public health organizations. Participants included individuals, the media, industry, non-profit-making organizations and national and local government.

essential factor in the success of these efforts is the dissemination of relevant knowledge throughout society. Towards that end, it has become indispensable to involve nongovernmental organizations and cooperate closely with the media.

To encourage public participation, policy-makers can:

- identify the various participants as representatives, to discourage them from allowing competitive, private, professional or corporate interests to cloud their contributions;

- make sure that the most vulnerable and least privileged population groups are proportionally and fairly represented in the consultation process;
- make sure that information – and its presentation – is objective and clear;
- express clearly from the beginning of the process the degree to which a public policy can realistically incorporate participant views; and
- provide feedback to the populace about the outcome of the consultation process and how it has been used.

How can policy-makers incorporate up-to-date data into their health policies?

Ethical governance in the health sector implies the continual collection and monitoring of data on population health, health risks and health determinants, which enable the health authorities to make decisions based on the latest facts and knowledge. Data collection is hardly a new tool for defining and implementing policies, but it continues to become more powerful as it is refined by experts. One such improvement is the collection of disaggregated data, which allow policy-makers to assess the distribution of health benefits among the different population groups – i.e. to make an equity analysis.

TOOL FOUR – Gather health data and develop health intelligence

For a health policy that seeks to be both practical (efficient and financially realistic) and ethical (responsive and value-driven), it is essential to monitor population health status closely. This necessitates the constant observation and interpretation of a broad set of health indicators (see Boxes 21–23).

In developing a permanent system of health indicators, policy-makers should ensure that it respects ethical norms, including the individual's right to privacy and lifestyle choice. In data collection and monitoring, that means that individual data should be anonymous and confidentiality strictly guaranteed.

BOX 21. DATA TOOLS DEVELOPED BY THE WHO REGIONAL OFFICE FOR EUROPE

The European health for all database consists of data on nearly 600 health indicators for each of the Region's 52 Member States. It is accessible at http://www.euro.who.int/hfadb.

Assorted technical databases (such as for tobacco consumption and communicable diseases) that enable international comparisons are also accessible on the Regional Office web site (http://www.euro.who.int).

The European health report is published periodically, summarizing the population health status and main health indicators for each Member State, and identifying fields for action. The report aims to supply decision-makers with current information that can be used directly. Some countries prepare their own national health reports for a similar purpose.

BOX 22. DATA TOOLS DEVELOPED BY OTHER ORGANIZATIONS

OECD health data are the largest statistical source for comparing health status among member countries of the OECD. This unique interactive database is a fundamental tool for health researchers and health policy advisers in government, the private sector and academia. It gathers in one place more than 1200 indicators, as well as the results of in-depth questionnaires.

"Key data on health" bring together information from a vast array of scientific sources and include data on health status and diseases, environmental and road hazards, and lifestyle factors, as well as the health care system itself. The report, assembled by Eurostat (the Statistical Office of the European Communities), is intended as a tool for EU health policy-makers, medical specialists, health economists and researchers, as well as members of the media and the general public.

Other EU bodies engaged in health data work include the EU Public Health Programme, which is actively developing health indicators under its Health Information Strand, and the Indicators Subgroup of the Social Protection Committee, which is also working with health indicators in order to supply better information for health service initiatives.

BOX 23. PROTOCOL ON WATER AND HEALTH

This protocol to the 1992 Convention on the Protection and Use of Transboundary Watercourses and International Lakes is a powerful mechanism for gathering health data. Adopted in 1999 at the Third Ministerial Conference on Environment and Health, the Protocol is also the first major international legal instrument for the prevention, control and reduction of water-related diseases in Europe. It entered into force in August 2005 and became legally binding on ratifying countries. At a meeting of the parties to the Protocol, quality data collection was recognized as essential to successful surveillance and the creation of effective reporting mechanisms.

TOOL FIVE – Develop and maintain health crisis monitoring systems

Health crisis monitoring systems are an essential tool used to anticipate catastrophic health emergencies when possible, and otherwise to respond to disasters as soon as they occur. While health alert systems primarily monitor infectious diseases, crisis monitoring systems have increasingly also begun to monitor major environmental health risks. Such systems have become indispensable in addressing disasters in an increasingly globalized world, where diseases spread with ever greater ease and rapidity.

Health crisis monitoring systems are useful because they can:

- detect major health threats and emergencies
- assemble current knowledge of health risks and assess it critically
- evaluate and analyse emergencies
- alert the authorities to potential major threats
- form a basis for both ad hoc and systemic recommendations
- bolster the crisis surveillance efforts of health care professionals.

For maximum effectiveness, such systems must draw on a network of national, regional and global partners. Rapid responses to disease outbreaks at the community level usually require a central team linked closely to local epidemiology units. The team should also be linked to a network of investigative epidemiology laboratories and a well-organized transport system.

The effectiveness of a health crisis monitoring system depends on its flexibility, its ability to detect unforeseen risks, the extent of its intersectoral coordination, its funding support, its independence from political authorities and agendas, and its communications capabilities.

The link to Health for All values

Often in an emergency, only collective action can ensure that vital protection measures are carried out for the benefit of the weakest and poorest (and thus for all). When epidemics occur, effective public health protection is guaranteed primarily by instituting measures for the entire population as quickly as possible and, if necessary, in an authoritarian manner. The implementation of such measures should nevertheless respect the principles of fairness and solidarity. International responses to health emergencies similarly need to show respect for these values (see Box 24).

BOX 24. WHO EFFORTS

The International Health Regulations were revised and adopted by the World Health Assembly in May 2005. The Regulations represent a major advance in protecting global health from disease risks, irrespective of their origin or source.

The Global Outbreak Alert and Response Network (GOARN) links experts, health care institutes and public health authorities. This electronic network has numerous components, including:

- the global public health information network – a worldwide database with a system-wide search engine, in which keywords may be entered in seven languages to identify the indicators of an epidemic outbreak; and
- the WHO network of laboratories – currently 110 laboratories in 84 countries.

GOARN enables WHO to react to crises in real time, issuing health warnings rapidly around the world, sending out information bulletins, advising individuals, developing crisis strategies and providing support for governmental actions. Its capacity was demonstrated during the SARS (severe acute respiratory syndrome) crisis.

TOOL SIX – Monitor health determinants

The United Nations Committee on Economic, Social and Cultural Rights interprets the right to health as an inclusive right that applies to health determinants as well as to health care. Accordingly, governments should strive to safeguard the individual's right not only to timely and appropriate health care, but also to safe and potable water, adequate sanitation, adequate supplies of safe food and nutrition, safe and adequate housing, healthy occupational and environmental conditions, and education and information on health topics, including sexual and reproductive health.

Deciding on and implementing health initiatives is most effective when based on a clear understanding of the major health determinants. Monitoring health determinants requires a coordinated approach both inside and outside the health sector. It is important that inequalities related to health determinants be monitored and presented in both relative and absolute terms. This approach is needed because interventions to reduce disease and save lives can succeed only when social determinants of health are adequately accounted for. Much has been learned about these determinants from national and international projects and studies, but the knowledge that has been gathered is still somewhat fragmentary. In order to be fully utilized, it needs to be more fully developed and widely disseminated.

That is why both the 2002 and 2003 editions of *The world health report* address the burden of disease *(48,49)*. The 2002 report is devoted to 10 risk factors – malnutrition, unsafe sexual practices, high blood pressure, tobacco use, alcohol use, unhealthy environments, iron deficiency, the burning of solid fuels and indoor air pollution, high cholesterol and obesity – and the burden of disease attributable to each one. Together, these 10 risk factors (which include lifestyle characteristics as well as health determinants) are responsible for more than a third of all deaths in the world.

The 2002 report also calculates how much disease, incapacity and death could be avoided during the next 20 years if appropriate measures were taken now to address these risks. It shows how significant gains in healthy life expectancy can be achieved in both the poorest and the richest countries in the next decade through relatively modest means. By adopting WHO risk assessment methods, a government can facilitate its efforts to reduce its national burden of disease and improve its population health.

The link to ethical governance
One of the most effective ways to deal with a widening gap in health status within a population is to target the social determinants of health, notably poverty. Such actions have the broader aim of improving the circumstances in which people live and work, which is of paramount importance in improving health and reducing health inequities. Since the major health determinants are themselves socially determined, at least in part, they also need to be addressed socially (see Box 25). The

Established in 2005, the Commission is the latest global effort by WHO to respond to the problem of social health determinants. One part of the Regional Office for Europe – the Venice-based European Office for Investment for Health and Development – seeks to bring together the concepts, scientific evidence, technology and policy actions needed to address the social and economic determinants of population health. In conjunction with the new Commission, the Venice office is working closely with European countries to expand activities in this area.

leadership needed to institute such remedies is accordingly located within public decision-making institutions that deal with social policy and action.

Not only do strategies that address basic health determinants have a positive impact on health; in general, they also promote sustainable development and reduce inequity. But to deal with health determinants, health policy often has to address personal and collective behaviours as well. In developing the health strategies to do so, a government should consider the ethical consequences and make sure that they respect personal rights and freedoms, especially when dealing with determinants that depend on individual behaviours. Deciding on the best way to address them may be difficult. Sometimes better results are achieved by using education instead of legal prohibition to change unhealthy behaviours. However, prohibitions can sometimes be effective, too. In France, for instance, a strategy of prohibitions and sanctions achieved a dramatic reduction in automobile accidents in 2002–2004, though the strategy's long-term sustainability has yet to be demonstrated.

How can health policy-makers assess the implementation of policy values?

TOOL SEVEN – Assess health system performance

WHO first began evaluating and analysing the performance of health systems in an attempt to understand the significant inequalities in health gains around the world. Abundant evidence had shown that comparable countries making similar investments sometimes obtained very different results in health improvement and that, conversely, different levels of investment sometimes produced similar results. This pattern raised questions about the efficiency of health systems – their ability to obtain for their money not only the best health outcomes, but also the maximum degree of responsiveness and of fairness in financing.

In *The world health report 2000*, WHO presents some analytical tools that illuminate health system weaknesses and help explain differences in health system performance *(50)*. These tools measure performance with respect to health system goals such as health gain, responsiveness and fairness. The report's findings include two observations that are particularly relevant to systems committed to Health for All.

- **The poverty trap**. The consequences of malfunctioning health systems are inversely proportional to income, being much greater in low-income countries. When a health system is not working properly, the gaps between rich and poor in low-income countries are also much greater in terms of patient dignity and patient choice. Such systems therefore do not fully respect their poorest users' right to health.

- **Fair financial contributions**. Health system costs should be shared fairly – which means that policy-makers should ensure that the poorest people do not devote a higher percentage of their revenue to protecting their health than the rich do.

Analysing health system performance has generated some interesting comparisons and triggered some important debates *(51)*. It is beneficial for a government to encourage such debates and delve into the causes of inequities, and it reflects a basic ethical commitment. Until now, however, this type of analysis has suffered from certain limitations in the sophistication of the indicators used and the quality of the information gathered. Future developments in the assessment of health system performance will require better tools. Nevertheless, assessing the performance of the health system is an important step in implementing Health for All values (see Box 26).

In 1999, WHO supported the creation of the Observatory to help the transition
countries in the European Region scrutinize how their health sectors were functioning
in comparison to each other and to western European models. The Observatory has
since undertaken numerous studies, including a series of national surveys that help
those responsible for health care to describe their own systems, using a common
scheme and methodology. These surveys provide a wealth of comparative data, which
health systems have found invaluable for all kinds of internal and collaborative analyses.

TOOL EIGHT – Assess quality: accreditation

Health care accreditation is a tool that can be applied at different levels.
On a national scale, it is an all-round tool used to ensure health care safety
and quality, and to encourage continual improvement. Accreditation is
also conducted in the individual health care setting by having external
professionals review its functioning and practices. They suggest how the
facility can strengthen the weak aspects of its organization, equipment
and operations and bring them up to established standards. These
standards have been developed by other health professionals, either
independently or in collaboration with a specialized independent body.

Accreditation confers a number of potential benefits. Quality and
safety of medical care are evaluated in relation to patient expectations.
Accreditation focuses on continual improvement in treatment and
diagnosis. Peer evaluators provide specific recommendations to
health care professionals on how they can bring performance up to
desired standards. Since fellow professionals are directly involved in
the accreditation process, those being evaluated therefore tend to be
more willing to accept and implement proposed changes. Because
assessments are conducted by outside experts, professionals and
patients alike can rely on them to make judgements that are objective
and informed. Accreditation reports are available to the general public,
increasing patient confidence.

It is important to note that accreditation is only one among a number
of tools for quality development and quality assurance; others include
clinical guidelines, quality recommendations and audits.

The link to Health for All values
Accreditation provides a government with an opportunity to formulate and promote quality standards in the common interest. It can also bring together and motivate health care professionals, and give members of the general public the information they need to compare provider options and choose well among them. In short, though it requires some investment of human and financial resources, accreditation can lead to greater access, broader participation and increased transparency (see Box 27).

BOX 27. THE EUROPEAN EXPERIENCE

The health sectors in Canada and the United States of America have been using accreditation systems for a long time. Since 1980, most European countries have experimented with the approach, though only a few have established permanent accreditation systems. The first attempt took place within the United Kingdom, though the system was never fully developed. The British model was later tested in Finland, Portugal and Sweden, where some voluntary accreditation systems of limited scope were developed. Some private establishments in the Czech Republic, Hungary, Poland, Portugal, Spain and Switzerland lobbied their respective governments to introduce accreditation, but other methods for improving quality of care were chosen instead. In Germany there is a voluntary certification procedure for hospitals, used to evaluate all medical and nursing care and administrative procedures. It is geared to the best international certification practices in health care and is implemented by accredited, decentralized organizations.

Today, only a few European countries accredit their health facilities and programmes. In Belgium, there exists a national accreditation system for laboratories. France has set up an accreditation agency, and all 3000 public and private medical establishments there must now undergo a quality and safety assessment carried out by specially trained external experts. Within the United Kingdom, Scotland is instituting separate accreditation schemes for some priority programmes, such as cancer, cardiovascular diseases and mental health. Although other countries in the European Region are committed to improving the clinical and organizational quality of their health systems, they have stayed away from accreditation thus far.

How can policy-makers further rationalize health policies and actions?

TOOL NINE – Base health policy on evidence
In this age of exponential growth in knowledge, health policies are increasingly taking account of scientific criteria and evidence. But

for decision-makers to maximize the effectiveness of health sector programmes, they need access to current data and the best evidence available. Current studies of how to base health policy on evidence have focused on refining the process and increasing applicability. Good health evidence includes not only research results but also other types of knowledge that decision-makers may find useful. Fortunately, there are now several excellent sources of ideas and information that are particularly targeted at health authorities (see Boxes 28–30).

BOX 28. THE COCHRANE COLLABORATION

This international organization produces systematic reviews of current medical literature on the effectiveness of particular health interventions. Health professionals, policy-makers and health care users all use these reviews, which are available to members at http://www.cochrane.org. Review abstracts are available on the site to everyone for free. The Collaboration has established specific protocols to minimize potential reviewer bias, including peer review. The organization also conducts in-depth methodological research summarizing scientific knowledge in medicine and health.

BOX 29. WHO REGIONAL OFFICE FOR EUROPE

The Health Evidence Network (HEN), an online information service developed by the Regional Office (http://www.euro.who.int/hen), is aimed primarily at health decision-makers in the public sector, although other parties also find its offerings useful. An international editorial staff discusses proposed questions, seeking topics that best reflect policy-makers' interests. Then an expert in the field synthesizes answers to each chosen question, drawing on a variety of documents, surveys and studies to describe the recent evidence, scientific and ethical dimensions, etc. All HEN synthesis reports are subjected to peer scrutiny and periodic updates. A handbook for evidence-based working and case-study writing is also available from the Regional Office.

BOX 30. INTERNATIONAL NETWORK OF AGENCIES FOR HEALTH TECHNOLOGY ASSESSMENT (INAHTA)

This network enables health technology assessment agencies and scientific societies to share methods and findings with each other. Linking 40 agencies from 20 countries, INAHTA also enables its members to pursue joint interests. Inasmuch as medical technology assessment is a multidisciplinary field within the domain of policy analysis, the Network serves as a forum for policy-makers too. Its web site (http://www.inahta.org) provides links to relevant databanks, newsletters and reports, while a comprehensive database covers both in-progress and published studies, with summaries and useful references.

The link to ethical governance
In the long run, choosing to ground policy in evidence can only bring health improvement – an idea that is admittedly much easier to proclaim than to put into practice. Even though scientific findings can provide a solid foundation for health policy decisions, evidence-based methods are not always easy to implement. Often, evidence for the health impact of a certain factor cannot be readily demonstrated when needed, owing to the complexity of various overlapping factors. And when it comes to new health hazards, reliable predictive studies are time-consuming and costly. Other recurrent problems include situations where evidence is clear but does not influence decision-making, or where decisions must be made but the necessary evidence is lacking. Establishing a fast link between policy and evidence can be a breakthrough in formulating enlightened health policy, in both the health sector and other sectors.

TOOL TEN – Conduct health impact assessments
Health impact assessment (HIA) is a set of methods and tools designed to incorporate a health dimension in all public policy. By means of HIA, a policy, programme or plan may be evaluated for its potential effects on health. Decisions made in sectors such as industry, transport, environment, housing, agriculture and energy have a variety of health consequences, direct or indirect. HIA tries to predict these effects beforehand, in order to inform decision-making, and it can therefore be an invaluable tool in introducing health considerations to non-health sectors (see Boxes 31 and 32).

HIA has proven to be an effective means of raising the profile of public health on the political agenda. Traditionally, policies in other sectors are developed with limited consideration for their health implications; yet when adverse health consequences arise, their costs are borne by the health sector. Involving the health sector in consultation on other sectors' policies and plans can help to anticipate such situations. For it to be effective, HIA should involve all relevant stakeholders, including the affected population, and participants should be willing to question the value of programmes that are shown to have a negative impact on public health. And for maximum effectiveness, HIA should also use the best available evidence on health and its determinants.

BOX 31. THE EUROPEAN EXPERIENCE

The EU first articulated the requirement that the formulation and implementation of all EU policies, programmes and activities must ensure a high degree of health protection in two foundational documents, the Treaty on European Union (Maastricht Treaty) and the Treaty of Amsterdam. Its Directorate-General for Health and Consumer Protection is charged with evaluating public health consequences for every EU policy and programme. The basis for integrating health considerations into other sectors' policies was established even earlier, with a 1985 directive that made environmental impact assessment obligatory for all EU Member States.

Various individual European governments have also instituted HIA provisions. Ireland, the Netherlands, Sweden and the United Kingdom have each developed a national system for evaluating the health impact of public policy actions and programmes. While HIA is not yet broadly used throughout Europe, many countries have implemented national, regional or local HIA projects that have advanced rapidly in recent years. Several European countries have also set up HIA pilot schemes and are testing various tools, including methodological guides, manuals, indicator lists, training courses and seminars. The core methodology is itself quite well defined, and good HIA information sources are also available, such as the Health Impact Assessment Gateway (http://www.hiagateway.org.uk) and the WHO HIA web site (http://www.who.int/hia).

BOX 32. EUROPEAN ENVIRONMENT AND HEALTH COMMITTEE

Formed in 1995, the Committee includes representatives of health ministries, environmental ministries and intergovernmental and nongovernmental organizations in the European Region. It acts as a discussion forum and steering committee for a conference of health and environment ministers that takes place every five years (the next is to be held in 2009). The Committee's primary mission is to ensure implementation of the Environmental Health Action Plan for Europe, which was adopted at the second such conference in 1994.

One difficulty in employing HIA is the potential for competition with the priorities of other social sectors (such as finance, development, housing and employment). The fact that the negative health consequences of many projects only appear in time heightens the difficulty. Nevertheless, some countries of the European Region have discovered that HIA can actually increase the interest and involvement of the population, the academic community and local authorities.

HIA methods are still in development, with specialists working to improve procedures and create a common set of reference standards and protocols.

7. The Health for All road: a checklist for policy-makers

In the Health for All concept, updating a policy is as important as its implementation and evaluation. For the health of a country's population, it is vital to conduct a regular "check-up" of the national health policy – a systematic, periodic review of its content and implementation, particularly with respect to progress on Health for All principles. Not only does such a check-up make it easier for the health sector to adopt new approaches, but it can also provide stakeholders with an updated picture of how their health system is functioning. Of course, a comprehensive review is more straightforward when national health targets have been actively developed and articulated.

Many national experts have expressed interest in learning more about how to assess the performance of their national health policies with respect to the European Region's Health for All policy framework. This chapter proposes a rough checklist for how to do that, in the form of open-ended questions that might be addressed in a systematic policy review. The list is not meant to be exhaustive; rather, it gives examples of the type of questions that national policy-makers might wish to pose. Like the toolbox in Chapter 6, the following checklist is meant to encourage creativity and choice, while providing policy-makers with a methodology that can facilitate comparisons among countries.

Does the national policy support the core Health for All values?

This update has focused on three core health policy values that promote health for all. Policy support for **equity** and **solidarity** can be evaluated by answering questions such as those below.

- Does every inhabitant have access to all health services? This question is particularly critical to ask about primary care settings and different geographical areas.
- How does the policy make sure that no inhabitant is excluded from the health system?
- How is equity in access to health services monitored? When inequities are recorded, what procedures are in place to turn the observations into appropriate action?
- Who are the primary users of existing health services? If a proportionally greater number of them are for instance wealthier inhabitants, then there are equity issues to resolve.
- Are there mechanisms to compensate for inequalities and support the most vulnerable groups? Possible approaches include disseminating targeted information to these groups and encouraging their use of existing services.
- Is there a national strategy for addressing health determinants? How does it try to ensure that the way these determinants impact the health of various population groups is equitable and fair?
- What is done to ensure that intersectoral cooperation does not undermine respect for equity in health policy?

Not only is consulting the public and other stakeholders an excellent source of new ideas, but such participation increases the sense of public ownership and shared responsibility for new initiatives. Moreover, it lends the health sector more popular authority in its interactions with other public sectors, such as finance, education, environment and justice. For **public participation**, then, the questions should focus more on policy and programme development.

- How receptive is the health system to public opinion? Do all members of the public have an equal opportunity to make their views known?
- What mechanisms are in place to encourage public participation? What is done to encourage the participation of members of disadvantaged and vulnerable groups?
- When major new health policies and programmes are being developed, are there ample opportunities for public discussion

and debate? Which major stakeholders are consulted? Which ones are not? Are these activities arranged in good time and publicized widely?

Does the policy reflect a broad vision of health?

A second critical aspect to examine in a health policy is whether the balance of components reflects the relative contributions they make to health. To evaluate this balance, another set of questions needs to be posed.

- What programmes and initiatives exist to promote healthy lifestyles? Are there national action plans for tobacco, alcohol, drug addiction, nutrition and physical activity?
- What are the criteria for evaluating whether health care services improve health? How can these criteria be made more effective?
- What programmes and initiatives exist to address environmental health? Is there a national action plan for environmental health?
- What programmes and initiatives exist to compensate for the impact of poverty on health? Is there a national action plan for poverty reduction?
- Of the four types of health programmes – patient care, prevention, promotion of healthy lifestyles and addressing health determinants – which has the greatest potential for improving population health? Which has the least? Do current budget allocations reflect these relative potentials? (For details on what each component includes, see pp. 14–16.)

A range of Regional Office documents in various technical areas – declarations, action plans, guidelines – is also available to help evaluate how well a national policy is balancing its obligations to address all the major health determinants.

How well does the health system reflect a commitment to Health for All?

Ultimately, what matters is whether Health for All values are put into practice. To evaluate implementation, one must examine several aspects of the health system to see how well it expresses these values.

(For a discussion of the health system's role in the pursuit of health for all, see pp. 17–18.) Again, as in the first group of questions (pp. 74–75), the question of access is central.

Quality improvement is another good indication that a health system is aligned with Health for All values.

- How does the system make sure that facilities perform to standard, both clinically and organizationally?
- How much training do health professionals receive in quality development?

Other areas of health system performance are also worth examining.

- How are health policy priorities established? What mechanisms help ensure that they are reflected in budget allocations?
- Are human resources distributed fairly among institutions and among geographical areas?
- Does health policy formulation draw on the experience of health professionals? Does it also draw on professional expertise from outside the health sector?

Health systems should be designed to minimize the inequities that stem from various social determinants. The way a health system is organized, financed and managed is itself a powerful determinant of health and health inequities. To evaluate how well a system addresses social determinants, several questions are germane.

- Is the national health system designed to minimize differences in access to care? Does it prevent inequities in the social consequences of ill health (such as disability and impoverishment)?
- Does the health system address the broader health determinants, such as poverty and educational level, through intersectoral planning and budgeting?
- How does the health system deal with discrepancies in the way certain diseases affect people from groups with different social positions or levels of vulnerability?

- Does the health system ensure members of vulnerable groups or groups with lower social positions equal opportunity in the use of health services, such as by defining priority health action zones or instituting positive discrimination schemes?

One interesting approach in analysing a national health system through the lens of ethical, values-based governance is to link the three general goals of all health systems – health improvement, fairness and responsiveness – to the Health for All values.

- Are health gains distributed with respect to the values of equity and solidarity?
- Are individual financial contributions to the system determined fairly? (Are contributions proportional to ability to pay?)
- Is the system responsive to the needs and vulnerabilities of all population groups, without discrimination?

Patient contributions are also worth inquiring about, especially when it comes to financing the health system.

- Are health system funds raised in a manner that distributes costs fairly?
- Are the funds pooled so that the entire population is guaranteed access to health services?
- When resources are allocated to health service providers, do the choices – what to buy, how much and for whom – reflect the values of equity and solidarity?

How do other factors influence the adoption and implementation of a Health for All policy?

In performing a health policy check-up, it can also be instructive to examine the factors that can affect the adoption and implementation of an explicit Health for All policy. These factors can be grouped into three categories: contents, process and context. A close look at these factors should precede any major Health for All reform, in order to increase the probability of its successful implementation, and it can thus provide a useful supplement to the questions above. Inasmuch as policy adoption and implementation processes are largely country-specific, this section focuses on the relevant policy content and context factors.

Analysing the contents of a Health for All policy

The nature of a Health for All policy makes it complex, if not difficult, to implement. While a number of factors facilitate implementation of the conventional health policy, few of them pertain to the Health for All policy. Table 2 should give policy-makers some insight into why a Health for All policy may be difficult to implement.

Table 2. How content-related factors affect health policy implementation

Characteristics of a conventional health policy that facilitate implementation	Corresponding characteristics of a Health for All policy
Simple technical features • Methods established and used widely • No new resources required	Highly complex technical features • Experience often lacking • Special training required • New information systems need to be developed
Marginal change from status quo • Incremental changes do not need approval or can be approved readily	Major shift from status quo • Major changes often strongly opposed by some stakeholders
Implementation by a single actor • No disagreements or compromises	Implementation by multiple actors • Typically multisectoral • Mix of private–public actors • Various levels often involved (from local to international)
Policy goals clearly stated • One main objective prevents confusion	Policy goals clearly stated • Goals may nonetheless be in conflict with other societal or health system goals
Rapidly implemented • Quick development process (which limits resistance and policy distortions)	Slowly implemented • Entire new system to painstakingly devise and initiate

Analysing the context: a Member State's capacity to absorb, adopt and implement a Health for All policy

Since the political context varies so greatly in the WHO European Region, the contextual factors that affect the implementation of a Health for All policy need to be addressed country by country. It may be helpful to consider the following questions in the light of national conditions.

What level of exposure do health policy actors have to the international exchange of health ideas, technologies and practices? Such exposure is particularly important in the public administration of health policy, and it contributes to the formation of international networks. Members of these networks, in which nongovernmental and international organizations play key roles, develop shared understandings of policy choices and problems.

What is the national capacity for health policy and health system research? This capacity cannot be taken for granted. For instance, while the demand for evidence-based health policies is growing, many countries are unable to satisfy it. To support the development and implementation of Health for All policies, many countries need to increase their capacity for such efforts.

Would the implementation of a Health for All policy be facilitated or hampered by the existing public health and health care infrastructure? For instance, is there an adequately trained health labour force? The content analysis in Table 2 suggests some of the demands that Health for All policies can place upon infrastructure. Again, suitable infrastructure cannot be taken for granted in every Member State in the Region.

Would the existing culture in the government health sector advance or retard the implementation of a Health for All policy? Some countries have a venerable tradition of health policy development and implementation, and they have tackled issues such as equity, healthy lifestyle promotion and multisectorality over a long period. Such a tradition may involve many societal systems, including the legislative and executive branches. In other countries, where health policy development and implementation have been largely confined to the health care system, the multisectoral approach needed to support a Health for All policy can seem unwieldy and strange.

Is the health sector's stewardship function well developed, so that it could shoulder the implementation of a national Health for All policy without difficulty? Firm exercise of stewardship, in which the health system demonstrates leadership and influence with respect to other societal systems, is frequently mentioned as an aid to effective policy development and implementation. Examples of stewardship – or its absence – were noted in the Health for All survey results from almost every Member State (see Chapter 4).

8. Conclusion

This update takes Health for All in Europe another step forward. Now it is adopted, the work will continue. We are no longer in a situation where one common prescriptive strategy can address the rapidly changing reality of every Member State. That is why the Regional Office for Europe has committed itself to an open-ended Health for All process, a process that will be continually enriched by a variety of national experiences and perspectives, as well as the ongoing input and work of the Regional Office. Consultation with the Member States has already generated some intriguing proposals that will be taken up during this open-ended process. Some of these ideas are:

- to explore further the financial dimension of implementing Health for All policies in the Member States;
- to scrutinize precisely how ethical, value-based governance relates to health system functioning;
- to study the impact of health determinants in non-health sectors;
- to monitor systematically the use and applicability of the Health for All model in individual countries;
- to develop concrete tools for comparative analysis of Health for All policies;
- to explore the connections between the Health for All policy framework and the core policies of other key international stakeholders in public health;
- to develop benchmarks for the progressive implementation of Health for All; and
- to develop a broad Health for All communications platform at regional, national and subnational levels.

References

1. Resolution EUR/RC48/R5: Health for all policy framework for the European Region for the 21st century. In: *Report of the forty-eighth session.* Copenhagen, WHO Regional Office for Europe, 1998 (EUR/RC48/REC/1; http://www.euro.who.int/document/rc48/ereport.pdf, accessed 6 June 2005).
2. HEALTH21 – *the health for all policy framework for the WHO European Region.* Copenhagen, WHO Regional Office for Europe, 1998 (European Health for All Series No. 6; http://www.who.dk/document/health21/wa540ga199heeng.pdf, accessed 7 June 2005).
3. Update of the regional health for all (HFA) policy framework. In: *Report of the third session of the Tenth Standing Committee of the Regional Committee for Europe.* Copenhagen, WHO Regional Office for Europe, 2003 (EUR/RC52/SC(3)/REP; http://www.euro.who.int/governance/scrc/20021210_1, accessed 7 June 2005).
4. *Update of the regional Health for All (HFA) policy framework.* Copenhagen, WHO Regional Office for Europe, 2003 (EUR/RC53/8; http://www.euro.who.int/governance/rc/rc53/20030626_1, accessed 7 June 2005).
5. Resolution EUR/RC53/R3: Update of the regional Health for All (HFA) policy framework. In: *Report of the fifty-third session.* Copenhagen, WHO Regional Office for Europe, 2003 (EUR/RC53/REC/1; http://www.euro.who.int/document/rc53/ereport/pdf, accessed 7 June 2005).
6. *Follow-up to previous sessions of the WHO Regional Committee for Europe.* Copenhagen, WHO Regional Office for Europe, 2003 (EUR/RC54/12; http://www.euro.who.int/governance/rc/rc54/20040629_1, accessed 7 June 2005).

7. *HEALTH21 – an introduction to the health for all policy framework for the WHO European Region.* Copenhagen, WHO Regional Office for Europe, 1998 (European Health for All Series No. 5; http://www.euro.who.int/aboutwho/policy/20011019_3, accessed 7 June 2005).

8. *The WHO Regional Office for Europe's Country Strategy: "Matching services to new needs".* Copenhagen, WHO Regional Office for Europe, 2000 (EUR/RC50/10; http://www.euro.who.int/governance/rc/rc50/20010919_14, accessed 7 June 2005).

9. *United Nations Millennium Development Goals.* New York, United Nations, 2000 (http://www.un.org/millenniumgoals/, accessed 7 June 2005).

10. Constitution of the World Health Organization. In: *Basic Documents.* Geneva, World Health Organization, 2005 (http://www.who.int/governance/en, accessed 7 June 2005)

11. Resolution WHA30.43: Technical cooperation. In: *Handbook of resolutions and decisions of the World Health Assembly and the Executive Board, Volume II, 1973–1984.* Geneva, World Health Organization, 1985 (http://www.who.int/governance/en, accessed 7 June 2005).

12. *Primary care: report of the International Conference on Primary Health Care, Alma-Ata, USSR, 6–12 September 1978.* Geneva, World Health Organization, 1978 (http://www.who.int/hpr/NPH/docs/declaration_almaata.pdf, accessed 7 June 2005).

13. Resolution WHA34.36: Global Strategy for Health for All by the Year 2000. In: *Handbook of resolutions and decisions of the World Health Assembly and the Executive Board, Volume II, 1973–1984.* Geneva, World Health Organization, 1985 (http://www.who.int/governance/en, accessed 7 June 2005).

14. Resolution WHA35.23: Plan of action for implementing the Global Strategy for Health for All by the Year 2000. In: *Handbook of resolutions and decisions of the World Health Assembly and the Executive Board, Volume II, 1973–1984.* Geneva, World Health Organization, 1985 (http://www.who.int/governance/en, accessed 7 June 2005).

15. Resolution WHA48.16: WHO response to global change: renewing the health-for-all strategy. In: *Forty-eighth World Health Assembly.*

Geneva, 1–12 May 1995. Resolutions and decisions, annexes. Geneva, World Health Organization, 1995 (WHA48/1995/REC/1; http://www.who.int/governance/en, accessed 7 June 2005).

16. Resolution WHA50.28: WHO reform: linking the renewed health-for-all strategy with the Tenth General Programme of Work, programme budgeting and evaluation. In: *Fiftieth World Health Assembly. Geneva, 5–14 May 1997. Resolutions and decisions, annexes.* Geneva, World Health Organization, 1997 (WHA50/1997/REC/1; http://www.who.int/governance/en, accessed 7 June 2005).

17. Resolution WHA51.7: Health-for-all policy for the twenty-first century. In: *Fifty-first World Health Assembly. Geneva, 11–16 May 1998. Resolutions and decisions, annexes.* Geneva, World Health Organization, 1998 (WHA51/1998/REC/1; http://www.who.int/governance/en, accessed 7 June 2005).

18. Resolution EUR/RC30/R8: Regional strategy for attaining health for all by the year 2000. In: *Handbook of resolutions and decisions of the Regional Committee for Europe, Volume I, 12th edition.* Copenhagen, WHO Regional Office for Europe, 1989.

19. Resolution EUR/RC34/R5: Implementation of the regional strategy for attaining health for all by the year 2000: European regional targets. In: *Handbook of resolutions and decisions of the Regional Committee for Europe, Volume I, 12th edition.* Copenhagen, WHO Regional Office for Europe, 1989 (http://www.who.dk/governance/resolutions/20011026_5, accessed 7 June 2005).

20. Resolution EUR/RC41/R5: Strategy for attaining health for all by the year 2000: updating of the regional health for all targets. In: *Handbook of resolutions and decisions of the Regional Committee for Europe, Volume II, 1st edition.* Copenhagen, WHO Regional Office for Europe, 1995 (http://www.who.dk/governance/resolutions/20011017_3, accessed 7 June 2005).

21. *The right to the highest attainable standard of health: substantive issues arising in the implementation of the International Covenant on Economic, Social and Cultural Rights.* Geneva, Committee on Economic, Social and Cultural Rights, 2000 (E/C.12/2000/4; http://cesr.org/generalcomment14, accessed 7 June 2005).

22. Health and Consumer Protection Directorate-General: public health [web site]. Luxembourg, European Commission, 2005

(http://www.europa.eu.int/comm/dgs/health_consumer/
publichealth.htm, accessed 7 June 2005).

23. *Health for all by the year 2000: the Finnish national strategy.*
    Helsinki, Ministry of Social Affairs and Health, 1987.

24. *Health for all by the year 2000: revised strategy for co-operation.*
    Helsinki, Ministry of Social Affairs and Health, 1993.

25. *Government resolution on the 2015 public health programme.*
    Helsinki, Ministry of Social Affairs and Health, 2001.

26. Department of Health. *The health of the nation: a strategy for
    health in England.* London, The Stationery Office, 1992.

27. Secretary of State for Health. *Saving lives: our healthier nation.*
    London, The Stationery Office, 1999.

28. Weber I et al. *Dringliche Gesundheitsprobleme der Bevölkerung in
    der Bundesrepublik Deutschland: Zahlen – Fakten – Perspektiven.*
    Baden-Baden, Nomos Verlagsgesellschaft, 1990.

29. Weber I, Meye MR, Flatten G. *Vorrangige Gesundheitsprobleme in
    den verschiedenen Lebensabschnitten: Zwischenbericht.* Cologne,
    Eigenverlag, 1987.

30. Gesellschaft für Versicherungswissenschaft und -gestaltung (GVG)
    e.V. *Gesundheitsziele.de: Forum zur Entwicklung und Umsetzung
    von Gesundheitszielen in Deutschland.* Berlin, Bundesministerium
    für Gesundheit und Soziale Sicherung, 2003.

31. *Stadtdiagnose. Gesundheitsbericht Hamburg.* Hamburg, Behörde
    für Arbeit, Gesundheit und Soziales (BAGS), Freie und Hansestadt
    Hamburg, 1992.

32. *Gesundheit von Kindern und Jugendlichen in Hamburg:
    Zwischenbilanz 1994.* Hamburg, Behörde für Arbeit Gesundheit
    und Soziales (BAGS), Freie und Hansestadt Hamburg, 1995.

33. Ministerium für Arbeit, Soziales und Gesundheit des Landes
    Nordrhein-Westfalen. *Zehn vorrangige Gesundheitsziele für NRW.*
    Bielefeld, LÖGD (Landesinstitut für den ÖGD des Landes NRW),
    1995.

34. Ministère des Affaires Sociales de la Santé et de la Ville, Haut
    Comité de la Santé Publique. *La santé en France: Rapport général.*
    Paris, la Documentation française, 1994.

35. *Prescriptions for a healthier Norway: a broad policy for public
    health.* Oslo, Ministry of Social Affairs, 2002 (Report No. 16

(2002–2003) to the Storting (short version); http://odin.dep.no/ archive/hdvedlegg/01/07/folke013.pdf, accessed 7 June 2005).

36. Danis M, Clancy C, Churchill LR, eds. *Ethical dimensions of health policy*. Oxford, Oxford University Press, 2002.

37. McKee M. Values and beliefs in Europe. In: Marinker M, ed. *Health targets in Europe: polity, progress and promise*. London, BMJ Publishing Group, 2002.

38. *The human rights, ethical and moral dimensions of health care: 120 case studies*. Strasbourg, Council of Europe, 1998.

39. Nygren-Krug H. *25 Questions & answers on health and human rights*. Geneva, World Health Organization, 2002 (Health and Human Rights Publication Series Issue No. 1; http://www.who.int/ hhr/activities/en/25_questions_hhr.pdf, accessed 7 June 2005).

40. Culyer AJ, Wagstaff A. Equity and equality in health and health care. *Journal of Health Economics*, 1993, 12(4):431–457.

41. Whitehead M. The concepts and principles of equity and health. *International Journal of Health Services*, 1992, 22(3):429–445.

42. *General Assembly Resolution A 217 (III). Universal Declaration of Human Rights*. New York, United Nations, 1948 (http://www. un.org/documents/ga/res/3/ares3.htm, accessed 7 June 2005).

43. Daniels N. Fair process in patient selection for antiretroviral treatment in WHO's goals of 3 by 5. *Lancet*, published online 19 May 2005 (http://www.thelancet.com/journals/lancet/article/ PIIS014067360566518X/fulltext, accessed 7 June 2005).

44. *Convention for the Protection of Human Rights and Fundamental Freedoms: as amended by Protocol No. 11*. Strasbourg, Council of Europe, 1998 (http://conventions.coe.int/treaty/en/treaties/ html/005.htm, accessed 7 June 2005).

45. *European Social Charter (revised)*. Strasbourg, Council of Europe, 1996 (http://conventions.coe.int/Treaty/en/Treaties/Html/163. htm, accessed 16 June 2005)

46. Consolidated Version of the Treaty Establishing the European Community. *Official Journal of the European Communities*, C325/35, 24 December 2002 (http://europa.eu.int/abc/obj/amst/ en, accessed 7 June 2005).

47. Charter of Fundamental Rights of the European Union. *Official Journal of the European Communities*, 2000/C 364/01,

18 December 2000 (http://europa.eu.int/comm/justice_home/unit/charte/index_en.html, accessed 7 June 2005).

48. *The world health report 2002 – Reducing risks, promoting healthy life.* Geneva, World Health Organization, 2002 (http://www.who.int/whr/2002/en/index.html, accessed 16 June 2005)

49. *The world health report 2003 – Shaping the future.* Geneva, World Health Organization, 2003 (http://www.who.int/whr/2003/en/index.html, accessed 16 June 2005)

50. *The world health report 2000 – Health systems: improving performance.* Geneva, World Health Organization, 2000 (http://www.who.int/whr/2000/en/index.html, accessed 16 June 2005).

51. Murray CJL, Evans DB, eds. *Health systems performance assessment: debates, methods and empiricism.* Geneva, World Health Organization, 2003.

Annex 1

Key policy documents of the
WHO Regional Committee for Europe relevant to
development of the Health for All process

2004

Towards a European strategy on noncommunicable diseases (EUR/RC54/8)

Partnerships for health: Collaboration within the United Nations system and with other intergovernmental and nongovernmental organizations (EUR/RC54/Inf.Doc./3)

2003

Mental health in WHO's European Region (EUR/RC53/7)

The health of children and adolescents in WHO's European Region (EUR/RC53/11)

2002

Partnerships for health (EUR/RC52/7)

Poverty and health – Evidence and action in WHO's European Region (EUR/RC52/8)

Tuberculosis, HIV/AIDS and malaria (EUR/RC52/9)

The role of the private sector and privatization in European health systems (EUR/RC52/10)

European Strategy for Tobacco Control (EUR/RC52/11)

Poverty and health – evidence and action in WHO's European Region (EUR/RC52/BD/1)

2001

Partnerships for health (EUR/RC51/6)

Poverty and health – Evidence and action in WHO's European Region (EUR/RC51/8)

2000

The impact of food and nutrition on public health (EUR/RC50/8)

Eradication of poliomyelitis in the European Region and plan of action for certification 2000–2003 (EUR/RC50/9)

The WHO Regional Office for Europe's Country Strategy "Matching services to new needs" (EUR/RC50/10)